"Your Body Already Knows – *an apt title indeed. In this book, Nidhi, a dedicated Ayurvedic healer, offers a profound response to the health concerns that plague modern society. Rather than treating symptoms in isolation, Nidhi takes each individual's unique health issues as her starting point, crafting a holistic approach rooted deeply in the science and wisdom of Ayurveda. Her explanations are anchored in traditional Ayurvedic principles yet remain accessible and relevant to today's world, making the profound essence of this ancient science resonate with our contemporary needs.*

As I read this work, I couldn't help but think of the Bhagavad Gita, where Sage Veda Vyasa guided a despairing Arjuna through his inner turmoil to a place of clarity and purpose. In a similar way, Your Body Already Knows *acts as a guide for those struggling in their personal health battles, offering reasoned advice grounded in timeless wisdom. Like Arjuna, many today find themselves disoriented and disconnected, unsure of how to move forward in a world filled with stress, anxiety, and seemingly insurmountable challenges. Nidhi's book is a gift to such a society – a beacon for those seeking not just to survive but to thrive with knowledge, awareness, and harmony.*

With this book, Nidhi provides a path forward, reconnecting readers with their innate ability to heal and achieve balance through the teachings of Ayurveda. It's a journey back to wholeness, reminding us that the wisdom we seek always lies within. Nidhi, your dedication and passion are evident in this masterpiece. I'm honored to wish you and your book all the success in the world. "

Guru Yogi Shivan,
Indimasi Healing Village, India

Praise for Your Body Already Knows

"Ayur means life. Ayurveda is the science of life. In its essence, life is a combination of a certain amount of time and energy. Hence Ayurveda is the science of maximizing time and energy to facilitate profoundness of human experience and impactfulness of one's activity. It is in making our body–mind structure into a stepping stone rather than an impediment that it becomes possible for an individual life to tap into the intelligence of the larger creation and the source of creation. Ayurveda is not just a health system but the science of exploring the human mechanism and consciousness in utmost profoundness, and that naturally involves a deeper understanding of all life upon the planet and its nature. Deeply appreciate Nidhi Bhanshali Pandya's efforts to bring the science of Ayurveda with a fresh look to the world."

– **Sadhguru**, founder of the Isha Foundation, author of the New York Times bestseller *Inner Engineering* and many other books

"Your Body Already Knows *is a succinct guide to anyone seeking an integrative approach to well-being at all levels – body, mind, and spirit.*"

– **Deepak Chopra MD**, world-renowned pioneer in integrative medicine, founder of the Chopra Foundation and New York Times bestselling author of over 90 books

"Ayurveda is the original lifestyle and personalized medicine, and it allows us to develop heightened awareness for intuitive healing. Nidhi Bhanshali Pandya has done an amazing job of presenting this ancient Ayurvedic wisdom for a modern audience."

– **Dr Suhas Kshirsagar BAMS MD (Ayu)**, author of
Change Your Schedule, Change Your Life

"Nidhi has a unique extraordinary gift for demystifying Ayurvedic concepts and presenting them in a clear and accessible way! Through insightful, patient references, she enriches the reader's understanding, making complex ideas feel relatable and practical. This engaging read invites you to explore the wisdom of Ayurveda, empowering you to integrate its principles into your everyday life."

– **Dr. Feby Maria Puravath Manikat, MD,**
Stanford Sleep Medicine

"A powerful compendium of theory and practice on how to move into genuine thriving, Dr. Nidhi's thoughtful teaching goes far beyond quick fixes. This jewel of a book presents lasting solutions for the most potent disease triggers of our time: generational trauma, weak genetic frameworks, and modern lifestyle habits that leave us stuck with more chronic health conditions than any generation before us. They are words of wisdom that empower you to unearth and heal the root causes of your disease by aligning with your body. *Your Body Already Knows* is a gem that I will keep on my nightstand and return to again and again!"

– **Anna Yusim, MD**, Clinical Assistant Professor,
Yale Medical School, and author of *Fulfilled*

"Birds fly south, whales migrate, and leaves fall with effortless ease. Our life too depends on living in sync with these invisible rhythms of nature. Your Body Already Knows will be your effortless guide, quietly whispering the wisdom of life through your thoughts, actions, and desires."

– **John Douillard DC, CAP**, author of seven books and founder of LifeSpa.com, where ancient Ayurvedic wisdom meets modern science

"I am so excited about this book! Nidhi has a gift for making epic, panoramic concepts accessible for all. We get to-the-point explanations of how Ayurveda's practices really work, and how to bring them into our lives without trying to do it all. Dive into this book if you've been looking for an empowering journey where you become your own healer."

–

Kate O'Donnell, author of The Everyday Ayurveda Cookbook and Everyday Ayurveda for Women's Health

"Nidhi is a master communicator of the ancient wisdom of Ayurveda. In this wonderfully straightforward and easy-to-follow book, she puts the management of health, along with the confidence and know-how, squarely in your hands. You will be able to kindle vibrant health, clarity, and spirit, through learning the basics of the cycles of the body and nature, and letting Ayurveda bring you in tune with them."

– **Eddie Stern**, creator of the Breathing App, yoga teacher, NYC, and author of One Simple Thing

Nidhi Bhanshali Pandya

Foreword by Jasmine Hemsley

YOUR

Body

ALREADY

Knows

Intuitive Ayurveda

21 Days to Reset your Gut, Sleep, Mood, and Health

WATKINS

Your Body Already Knows
Nidhi Bhanshali Pandya

This edition first published in the UK and USA in 2025 by
Watkins, an imprint of Watkins Media Limited
Unit 11, Shepperton House
89-93 Shepperton Road
London, N1 3DF

enquiries@watkinspublishing.com

2 3 4 5 6 7 8 9 10

Typeset by JCS Publishing Ltd.
Printed and bound by CPI Group (UK) Ltd, Croydon, CR0 4YY

The manufacturer's authorised representative in the EU for product safety is
eucomply OÜ - Pärnu mnt 139b-14, 11317 Tallinn, Estonia,
hello@eucompliancepartner.com,www.eucompliancepartner.com

A CIP record for this book is available from the British Library

ISBN: 978-1-78678-928-0 (Hardback)
ISBN: 978-1-78678-929-7 (eBook)

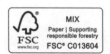

www.watkinspublishing.com

Thank you, Bapuji, my grandfather,
for leaving footprints in the sand

CO...

CONTENTS

FOREWORD

BY JASMINE HEMSLEY

Your Body Already Knows puts you back in the driver's seat when it comes to your mind–body health. It offers you the opportunity to reconnect with ancient and universal wisdom – wisdom that might well be intuitive had we not become so detached from nature, and our own inner nature. As Nidhi explains, "loss of wisdom" is, according to Ayurvedic texts, the main cause of all disease. How hard hitting is that, in this "Age of Information", when we are living at what we think of as the pinnacle of science, yet disease is more prevalent than ever!

The title of this book – *Your Body Already Knows* – makes me exhale in relief. It's a timely reminder that we can work with our body's innate wisdom and that overall wellbeing is within reach and should be nurtured by ourselves first and foremost.

As many do these days, Nidhi and I first connected online. I discovered her work through Instagram as I was researching Ayurvedic enthusiasts around the world to build my own community. At the same time Nidhi reached out to me, introducing herself, looking to make the science of life more accessible in the West. Before I knew it, we were swapping life stories, and she was bolstering me through a rather intense period of life as I embarked on the journey of pregnancy with my daughter Mahi. We swapped humorous and horrifying stories of morning sickness and other pregnancy mishaps, and she also shared Ayurvedic wisdom to inspire me physically, mentally and spiritually. Over the years she has become a great friend, always on the other end of WhatsApp voicenotes, ready to answer my Ayurvedic queries and help me connect the dots.

This book offers everything you need to immerse yourself in the knowledge of Ayurveda as a beginner and so much more for whom this book isn't your first Ayurvedic rodeo. It includes practical steps to build your awareness of how nature works and how imbalance affects your inner world. It encourages you to fine-tune yourself and nurture that inner knowing so you can begin to recognize when the mind–body needs a little attention. This is what I love about learning Ayurveda – those aha! moments become intuitive practices.

I wish I'd had access to this book when I first came to Ayurveda out of desperation in my 20s, when I was suffering chronic acid reflux, despite my apparently "healthy lifestyle". I was a little reluctant – how could ancient wisdom have much relevance in today's world, and if Ayurveda really worked, why wasn't it being implemented everywhere? However, when I experienced almost overnight relief after six months of getting no results from conventional meditation, I was hooked! With a few lifestyle adjustments, I managed to get rid of the acid reflux for good (it didn't even come back during my two pregnancies 15 or so years later).

With this book in your hands, you can implement Ayurvedic wisdom in just 21 days. Concentrating on just one new thing a day that you can incorporate into your life for long-term health gains feels very doable. With some of these practices you might notice almost immediate improvements in your digestion, mood and sleep, while other changes may be more subtle. In time you will experience the power of doing a daily practice in a non-rigid way, and realize how much easier life is when you go with the flow of the natural rhythms of nature – and how much more difficult life feels when you are swimming against it. This book makes the Ayurvedic lifestyle so much more sustainable in the long term.

As the business of wellbeing continues to explode, *Your Body Already Knows* reveals how many of the "new" trends and buzzwords, such as "circadian rhythm" (and by the way I love how Nidhi explains this as broken down into solar and lunar experiences), "internal body clock", "biohacks" etc, are actually based on Ayurveda's ancient understanding of health. By keeping the language universal, rather than requiring her readers to engage with Sanskrit (India's rich and complex ancient language), Nidhi makes this "new" way of understanding ourselves and our connection with nature completely accessible.

With this book, Ayurveda just makes sense. It makes sense because we are sensual beings interconnected with nature and its rhythms, and our health is linked to that of our immediate environment and ecosystem. As the macro, so the micro. Thank you, Nidhi, for reminding us of our innate wisdom, restoring our faith in our own abilities and helping us nurture a better relationship with our mind–body, and in turn with the world around us.

Jasmine Hemsley
Chef, well-being expert
and author of *East by West*

INTRODUCTION

Fortunately, Maha had the resources to consult the best experts for her many health matters. Unfortunately, she was emotionally and physically spent. After four long years of fertility treatments and a 16-year rollercoaster with eczema, she was exhausted. The bloating, painful periods, brittle hair, and constant anxiety – once her biggest concerns – had become part of the background noise of her life. She has mastered temporary fixes and even learned how to get through the day. But, by the time she came to me, something shifted. She was done with surviving. She wanted to wake up every day feeling truly alive, vibrant, and at ease in both her body and her mind.

Maha's story is not unique. I have heard countless others from around the world echo her words.

They all share a common desire: to stop treating and start healing.

Today, we have more wellness information at our fingertips than our grandparents ever did, yet we are more confused and disconnected than ever. Our minds and bodies are burdened with more debris than we can process – carrying generational trauma, weak genetic frameworks, and modern lifestyle habits that leave us stuck in a wellness matrix filled with endless suggestions but no real solutions.

But it doesn't have to be this way. You don't need a million answers to solve your million problems. The truth is, your body and mind are not separate: what heals one can heal the other. Your "dis-ease" doesn't need to evolve into disease. It can be your gateway to vibrant health – a powerful opportunity to undo, reset, and reclaim your true self.

Because life wants life.

Over the years, I've helped hundreds step into their healing and reclaim their power simply by tapping into what their bodies already know. You have that wisdom within you, too. All you need is the right guide to help you unlock it.

* * *

The Backstory

It was 1am when I heard footsteps in the corridor and looked up from my screen for the first time in hours. Three days earlier, my talk on Ayurveda had been a huge hit, and afterwards curious Mumbaiites had started to contact me, wanting to get personal with this timeless science of life, which originated in India 5,000 years ago. Since the event, some 50 people had lined up outside my office door, seeking an Ayurvedic verdict on their well-being. Left without much choice in the matter, I'd found myself sitting up into the small hours of the night to write mind–body assessments and recommendations for them all before I left for New York the next day.

Mom walked in to check on me, concerned about my well-being as I sat there still working to improve that of others. After expressing her perturbation, she made room for some pride. She poured water from the ceramic jug that sat neglected on the table before me and said, "You must be so fulfilled with your work. All your life, you've studied what makes people sick and what makes them tick. And here you are, a sought-after Ayurvedic expert. Your grandfather would have been so proud of you." Although I agreed with a smile, I knew that even in my tired state I was lying, more to myself than to her.

Fewer than 24 hours later, I caught the long-haul flight from Mumbai to New York. If you'd been a fellow passenger, you'd probably have concluded that I was squirming in my seat from the discomfort of being squished between my two daughters, but that would have been wrong. My restlessness was due to the dilemma that had surfaced with Mom's words of praise. Was I really fulfilled? Did I want to be the expert? I had dedicated a lifetime to understanding and studying how people, especially women, could live happier and healthier lives so that I could teach others and lighten their suffering. But while I had been able to help my clients find ease in their bodies in the short term, I felt that I'd taken away their power in the long term. Instead, I had set them up for dependency and despair.

After completing my Ayurveda education, I'd been thrust into a world where Ayurvedic practice mirrored modern-day medicine and took a prescription-based approach in which Ayurvedic doctors wrote up lists of do's and don'ts, and prescribed herbs and practices that offered their desperate clients a rigid new regimen, yet left them devoid of the principles behind it. After feeling better temporarily, most clients eventually either reverted to some version of their previous life, or continued their quest for yet more new experts and prescriptions, never truly grasping the root cause of their imbalance or how Ayurveda had initially intervened in it. They remained disempowered, lacking the understanding and confidence to care for their own well-being, and trapped in a cycle of fear, misinformation, and vulnerability within the bustling commercial wellness marketplace, where every other voice touts a quick-fix solution.

But let's set the record straight. Formal Ayurvedic treatments can indeed be transformative, offering solutions to chronic issues that have plagued individuals for years. Yet the crux of the problem from my perspective still lies in our tendency to relinquish all decision-making to experts. In today's world, experts abound, each challenging the previous one, leading to a never-ending cycle of perspectives. Sure, relying on an expert may initially provide a sense of security – after all, they usually know more than we do. But what happens to our autonomy over a lifetime of dependence? I've witnessed first-hand the anguish and turmoil experienced by those who incessantly seek out experts. They amass vast amounts of information but gain little true knowledge; they lack a synthesis of information, experience, and wisdom.

It's no surprise to me that age-old Ayurvedic texts list **Pragnya-aparadha,** or **loss of wisdom,** as the main cause of all diseases. Likewise, it wouldn't be surprising if our expert-led medical system is making us sicker. And the sick are constantly on the hunt for the next best thing in diets, exercise, and wellness trends; they unwittingly turn their bodies into testing grounds for marketers. Caught in a never-ending cycle of decision-making dilemmas and FOMO, they find themselves in a state of constant flux, disconnected from their bodies and far from the Ayurvedic ideal of health or *swasth*, which means **feeling steady in both body and mind.** *Swasth* is about finding healing, not treatment.

So no, I didn't want to be yet another "expert." This book is the result of what unfolded on that long, uncomfortable flight. It's the result of my wish to surrender my expertise so you can become your own expert and trust what your body already knows. But for that to happen, I will first have to introduce you briefly to Ayurveda, which underpins this book.

Ayurveda as a Way of Life

Ayurveda (*Ayuh*: life, *Veda*: science) is a science for living that originated in India in about 3000 BCE. Often dismissed by some as ancient, Ayurveda is in fact timeless and universal.

As long as the Earth revolves around the sun and rotates on its axis, Ayurveda will be relevant.

Ayurveda is also referred to as the sister science of yoga, as they both emerged from the broader Vedic systems of knowledge. Being the science of life, the scope of Ayurveda is extremely vast in its own right and covers everything from the prevention of disease, to nutrition, fertility, childcare, haircare, skincare, mental health, social conduct, and a lot more. If it has to do with human life, Ayurveda covers it. In fact, several recent trends like intermittent fasting, breathwork, bulletproof coffee (also known as butter coffee, made with added fat), turmeric, ashwagandha (used in herbal medicine), and the practices of oil swishing (also called oil pulling) and dry scrubbing have their origins in Ayurveda.

However, Ayurveda has never been just a subject to me; it was the language of my upbringing. Growing up in a sprawling extended family steeped in the Ayurvedic tradition, I absorbed its principles and practices as naturally as I breathed. My grandfather, a revered Ayurvedic healer, infused our daily lives with his wisdom, seamlessly weaving Ayurvedic insights into conversations without the need for formal declarations like "according to Ayurveda." Instead, his Ayurvedic teachings were intertwined with daily experiences, rooted in logic, connection, and intuition. Phrases like "beans are heavy to digest after sunset" or "your Agni [metabolic strength] is strong now; indulge if you must in the daytime" were common refrains, guiding our everyday choices with practical wisdom. For me, Ayurveda wasn't just a set of rules but a living, breathing philosophy passed down through generations. And as I embarked on my formal Ayurvedic education, I knew in my heart that I wanted to share this rich heritage with others, not just as a curriculum but as a way of life, grounded in the same intuitive wisdom that had shaped my own upbringing. The eternal optimist in me knew that this was possible.

The creatures of the natural world fueled my hope further. While nonintellectual in some respects, they were still connected to the body's intelligence, which guided them on how to live and eat. For example, deer don't need to consult a nutrition expert to know that a plant-based diet is best for them, nor do nocturnal tigers get carried away with the supposed health benefits of waking up early in the morning. They trust what their body already knows. As babies, we too are born with the innate sense that our mother's breast holds our food and that we need to use our mouth to access it, even though our existence in the womb is nil by mouth. No overthinking is involved, yet as we develop our intellect, we lose this connection, this intuition. I believed there had to be a way to return home to this inner wisdom so we could rediscover ourselves confidently so that we didn't always have to rely upon someone else to know what we need.

The Three Core Principles

I found my answer in the Vedas, the 5000-year-old scriptures from India, which are Ayurveda's parent texts. The Vedas contain profound truths about the realms that lie outside and within us, with guidance on how to navigate both. Some connective power allowed the ancient scientists to discover truths that we are still barely beginning to fathom today in our state-of-the-art laboratories. This verse from the *Yajur Veda* reveals their secret: *"Yatha pinde tatha brahmande, yatha brahmande tatha pinde"* – "As is the universe, so is the human body, and as is the human body, so is the universe."

The patterns of the universe hold clues to our own body's secrets, and vice versa. However, we can access these clues not through modern-day scientific equipment but through our keen awareness. The Vedic scientists were able to uncover subtle truths by quietening their minds so that they could use their awareness to decipher the hidden patterns of life. The process enabled them to uncover the truths of the planet and of our bodies, layer by layer.

I became even more determined to investigate. I paused my consumption of additional Ayurveda information and, instead, took what I already knew and began to explore it even more deeply to find the common threads. I wanted to be like Newton under that tree, watching the apple fall, or Archimedes in his bath tub, seeing objects sink and float. I wanted to learn from what I observed in the patterns of the universe. I began to have my own "aha" moments, too, which have never ceased to occur since then.

Over a period of time, what unfolded for me were three core principles that apply to everything on the planet, including how we eat, live, sleep, love, and feel. When I reopened my Ayurvedic ancient texts, I realized that, even though these principles weren't articulated as such, they were still to be found everywhere, between each line, in each concept and in every single recommendation. Once I had seen them, I couldn't unsee them – a bit like a puzzle that you struggle to solve, but once you do, you wonder how you ever missed the solution in the first place.

This book focuses on these three core principles, used by the original Ayurvedic scientists to decipher how life thrives, and will teach you how to apply them to every aspect of your life so you can become your own expert and thrive too.

How to Work with this Book

I want you to have what I have found: the ability to awaken the intelligence you already possess, reclaim your power and feel confident about being the driving force on your journey to health and happiness.

Even though I have always been magnetically drawn to Sanskrit, the language of the original Ayurvedic literature,

I'll be keeping the terminology in these pages to a minimum in order to make Ayurveda accessible to all. However, while the intention is not to go into all the detailed theories and different practices of Ayurveda, there are two profound concepts that are globally popular amongst the wellness-seeking population which do deserve their rightful place in this book:

- **Agni:** The Sanskrit word for fire, Agni is the term used for the warm digestive environment. In its use of it, Ayurveda may have been one of the first systems to talk about the importance of gut health.

- **The three doshas:** Embodying the idea of bio-individuality that draws many to Ayurveda, the concept of the three doshas classifies people according to the energy patterns of their body's inherent tendencies. Understanding bio-individuality can help us to be aware of our sensitivities, vulnerabilities, strengths, and weakness at both a physical and an emotional level, making it easier for us to navigate through life.

Your Body Already Knows doesn't obsess about these concepts, but breaks them down to make them more comprehensible. In particular, it explores them in the context of three core principles, and unfolds across four parts:

- In Part 1, "The Three Core Principles," I introduce you to three fundamental principles that will serve as your compass in understanding both yourself and the world. I will invite you to dive deep into each principle, letting them sink in slowly. You will discover how to train your awareness to discern these patterns in your daily life, empowering you to become a master pattern-seer, capable of not just observing but foreseeing trends in your life.

- Next, Part 2, "Living Ayurveda," will encourage you to immerse yourself in the application of these principles to key areas of your life, from diet and exercise to your mindset and relationships. Treat this part of the book as your training ground, where you learn to integrate the three core principles seamlessly into your daily routine. You needn't rush to enact every change immediately; instead, cultivate a vigilant awareness as everything falls into place.

- Part 3, "The Principles in Practice," thrusts you into the battlefield of daily practice. Over 21 days, I'll walk you through implementing the principles, one daily shift at a time. This timeframe is pivotal, allowing new habits to take root and patterns to undergo transformation. By introducing changes gradually, you can assimilate Ayurvedic wisdom steadily, ensuring sustainable growth.

- Finally, as you delve deeper into the three core principles and apply them to your life, you'll inevitably encounter questions, such as, "How do these principles adapt to life's different phases and external seasons?" Part 4, "Ayurveda for Life," addresses these queries and will show you how to embed the principles into your every-day existence, particularly in the most important areas.

My hope is that by the end of *Your Body Already Knows*, you will understand more Ayurveda than those who have studied Ayurveda academically for years, but through the use of your logic and intuitive wisdom. You will have more power over your wellness than the experts you've relied on thus far. And you will be left in awe as you tap in to what your body already knows.

If you already practice Ayurveda, it will take you beyond the rigid academic aspects of your practice and help you to connect with the wisdom at its roots, so you can make this more accessible for yourself and your clients. If you are a budding Ayurveda enthusiast, this book will cut through all the jargon and weave the nuanced science of life into your system like a first language. And if learning about Ayurveda isn't the main reason you picked up this book, even better: You have nothing to unlearn.

I have written this book for you, no matter who you are. I know that your body knows; this book is your first step in awakening its innate intelligence through the three guiding principles so that you can map a path to navigate through all areas of life. This will enable you to exit the cacophonous health market with its wellness trends and superficial quick fixes, and rediscover a source of inner trust within. As you'll see, Ayurveda has so much to offer those who live with Western medicine, as the two approaches are complementary and compatible. That said, if you have any medical concerns or suffer from health conditions, then do consult your medical practitioner before making any major lifestyle changes.

While the book is intended to be an easy read, it is not meant to be a quick read. Take a moment to grasp that. You may be tempted to go through it very quickly, but resist that urge. Sit with each concept. Go deeper, not wider. It's all within you anyway.

PART 1
THE THREE CORE PRINCIPLES

In the pages that follow, I am going to be sharing with you the three core principles that have become my lens through which I now explore and understand the patterns of the world and of human bodies and minds. It's how I study and teach Ayurveda. From being lost in the world, they have brought me to a place of endless wonder, allowing me to live in flow both within and outside myself, and to help hundreds of others to do the same.

These are the principles of:

- the Inner Climate® (a previously undefined concept, whose name I have now registered)

- the circadian rhythms

- the cycle of growth, transformation, and decline.

Once you get to know these principles and apply them, I'm confident that they will transform your life too.

THE INNER CLIMATE®

Life thrives in the optimum Inner Climate®. Our job is to notice when we deviate from it and find our way back each time.

Climate change is as real inside the human body as it is on our planet. You don't have to be a farmer to know that even the slightest change in climate can affect a crop's life; that if, for example, it snows in spring, there's a reason for this being labeled "freak weather." Unpredictable climate patterns are premonitory signs of an imbalance in life on Earth. A supportive environment led our planet, and it alone, to become home to 8.7 million species in over 4.5 billion years. Can you imagine what systematic climate change is doing now to all its inhabitants?

Similarly, imagine your body as a vast universe that is home to trillions of bacteria, which form a powerhouse called the microbiome. Just like every species needs a particular environment or climate in which to thrive, so does this inner army. Your inner army is a mighty force that helps you to digest your food, regulate your immune system, protect against bacteria that cause disease, and produce vitamins, including the B vitamins cobalamin, thiamin, and riboflavin, and vitamin K, which is needed for blood coagulation.[1] What is truly mind-blowing is that our microbiome actually provides more genes that contribute to human survival than the human genome itself (8 million as opposed to 22,000).[2] Without a healthy inner army of bacteria, our chances of thriving significantly plummet. Our Inner Climate® needs a certain type of climate if it is to be healthy. To put it simply:

Inner Climate® suffers = our inner army suffers = our body suffers

Picture this: when the Inner Climate® of your body is disturbed, this directly impacts the life of your microbiome and, consequently, your own life. It's a dynamic relationship that underscores the importance of nurturing this internal ecosystem for your overall well-being and vitality.

Just What is the Inner Climate®?

The ideal Inner Climate® inside the human body is warm and moist. This is the perfect state that allows life within us and thus our own life to thrive. Any deviation from this can lead to disease. Now, indulge me for a moment. Take your palms and cup them around your mouth; let out a large exhale till you can feel your breath in your palms. It will be warm and moist. As warm-blooded mammals, our blood is warm and moist, and so is our mother's milk. So are our reproductive fluids and urine. If you were to urinate one day and your urine seemed hotter than usual, this would instantly draw your attention as being something out of the ordinary. No wonder the first sign of severe sickness for most people is a fever, when the body quickly declares an emergency, taking it away from a lovingly warm to an alarmingly hot state.

Let me elaborate a little by drawing an analogy between our microbiome, which contains microbiota, also known as gut flora, and the general categories of flora and fauna. Where do flora and fauna thrive? The answer is in any warm and moist place – like Florida, which is particularly rich in animal and plant life. Yet its ecosystem could quickly become a breeding ground for parasites and mold as well, if it were overly humid and hot, like the Amazon rainforest. Too hot and dry, and the chances of survival dwindle, as they do in a desert. Cold like the Antarctic – forget it. Our microbiome and indeed our life itself thrive in warm and moist conditions, inside and out.

Now, let's delve deeper. We instinctively gravitate toward warm people, having an unspoken understanding of their intrinsic warmth. In contrast, coldness creates distance and renders relationships stagnant; at the other extreme, hot-tempered people burn through their social circles in no time. Not only a state of connection but even a state of flow becomes possible when our minds can bask in conditions of warmth and moisture.

Think for a moment about how you like your home environment to feel. I'm guessing it's neither too cold nor too hot. The fact is, no one much enjoys a sticky, humid room or a space that feels overly dry. Most of us prefer our surroundings to be comfortably warm and moist – just right, like our comfort foods, soups, and stews. Or like the comfort of a cozy blanket.

Just as we seek moisture and warmth, so does our inner army of gut microbiota and the planet itself – where the moon's moist and cool aspects balance the sun's heating and drying qualities. It is where almost all life exists and where life itself continues to thrive.

Our main job in Ayurveda is to return to and maintain an ideal Inner Climate®, to create an environment where life naturally thrives and sustains yet more life, and where our inner army is healthy enough to take on any battle and thus homeostasis becomes effortless. Once achieved, this means that we no longer have to dissect the needs of our body down to which micronutrients to consume or strive to achieve balance organ by organ, and system by system. We can finally liberate ourselves from the fear of disease and live in the freedom of good health. The yogis and Ayurvedic sages understood this truth, practiced it and used it to live in harmony with their bodies and minds for many long years.

I appreciate that it may seem more complicated to practice this concept than it is to understand it. If it's new to you, take a while to let it sink into your mind before trying to use it to change your life. After all, most of us have strayed away from the ideal warm and moist Inner Climate®. Almost every day, I meet people who are either too hot and inflamed, dry from depletion and exertion, or just stagnant, heavy, and humid due to immobility and over-nourishment. However, within three to four weeks of systematically incorporating the three principles that we'll be considering in these pages, they begin to heal and find their way back home in their bodies.

Throughout this book, I will teach you how your Inner Climate® can be rebalanced and enhanced with the integration of the two additional principles. I will then take you through a systematic journey in Part 3 that will enable you to restore your warm and moist Inner Climate® in 21 days.

Applying the Inner Climate® Perspective to the Ayurvedic Doshas

If this is not your first encounter with Ayurveda, there's a high probability that you've become enamored with the idea of the three doshas, kapha, pitta, and vata, and are invested in exploring your own doshic dominance. The doshas are three governing forces inside the body that guide all its physiological and psychological functions. The dosha that is the strongest in your body will determine your bio-individuality or doshic dominance. Ideally, all three doshas should be in balance, as doshic imbalance lies at the root of every disease.

If you're not especially into Ayurveda, feel free to skip this section altogether and move on to Principle 2 on page 22.

For those lovers of Ayurveda out there, let's do a dosha breakdown, but one that may be slightly different from what you're used to.

The Kapha Dosha

Kapha elements are protective and support the body in building volume and creating a system for its defense. They are pro-life; their properties are thick, cool, heavy, and slimy. Keep visualizing these thick and slimy properties as you continue reading...

Cytoplasm, the jelly-like substance that makes up the bulk of our cells and allows a cell's organelles (the substructures inside the cell) to stay safe, is kapha. The mucus lining that protects our insides from the body's warm juices and corrosive materials is another example of kapha. Similarly, the lymph that carefully carries immune cells throughout the body is kapha. The synovial fluid that forms the padding in the joints is kapha, too. So is the saliva in your mouth, the semen that carries the sperm and the cerebrospinal fluid that provides support and buoyancy to the brain – all kapha. Without kapha elements, we wouldn't be able to build new cells and would eventually wither away; nor would we be able to protect ourselves from our own warm blood.

Think of it like this: All the anabolic forces in the body join hands to form what we call the kapha dosha, yet we don't want our bodies to be dominated exclusively by kapha elements. If that were the case, we would build more than we need to, our bodies would become voluminous, slow and sluggish, our blood would accumulate plaque and slime, and our Inner Climate® would be far from warm and moist, deviating toward the humid, stagnant, and cold. A person who is kapha dominant can probably relate to this.

The Pitta Dosha

All the metabolic forces in the body join hands to form the pitta dosha. The pitta dosha, which is primarily hot and slightly moist, is responsible for the body's essential transformation and breakdown functions. It might help to visualize pitta as hot, thick oil as you read.

The digestive system is a pitta storehouse: Our digestive enzymes and bile are pitta elements that enable the breakdown and absorption of food. Pitta elements are also visible in the reproductive hormones and the ability to conceive. Pitta helps the nervous system to absorb sensory input and transform it into thoughts. It is likewise present in mitochondria, the powerhouse of each cell. The pitta dosha brings focus and passion. Without pitta, we would be lifeless, incapable, and stagnant beings. We wouldn't be able to digest our food or procreate, and our species would become extinct.

But we don't want the pitta dosha to take over the body. That would lead to severe inflammation, anger, and even burnout. Our food would liquefy and be evacuated before we could absorb its nutrients, and sperm would burn itself out before it could make its way to the ovum. We would be perpetually wired and exhausted, living in a chronic action and thinking mode. Our Inner Climate® would become overly hot and humid, and infections would make their home in our bodies. If the words "inflammation" or "burnout" are constantly at the top of your list of symptoms, you can probably relate to this.

The Vata Dosha

All the catabolic and mobile forces join hands to form the vata dosha. The vata dosha is the subtle force that allows for any type of movement in the body and for eventually drying and evacuating all that does not serve a purpose within. Try visualizing vata as a wind, gentle when its role is to move, and as a sharp gust when it seeks to dry and evacuate.

The vata dosha is responsible for our inhalations and exhalations. Similarly, it supports our body, allowing food to make its way down our gullet slowly and progress through the body until the waste matter is eventually expelled from the anus with its force. Vata is what allows the blood to defy gravity and move upward to replenish each and every cell of the body. It is this dosha that helps us to push and deliver a baby. Finally, in the last few years of our lives, it is vata that takes our force from us, dries our juices and depletes us, then leaves the body to face its demise.

Without vata, we would be immobile, breath-devoid beings. Our blood wouldn't circulate, and our bowels wouldn't evacuate themselves. Debris and dead cellular matter would remain within us, and our insides would rot. We wouldn't be able to fight or take flight when necessary. We would become inanimate.

It is evident, though, that we don't want vata to dominate. That would lead us to wither away, shrivel, and die before we could serve our purpose on this planet. Those in which vata is dominant are often dry, depleted, and scattered individuals. They may suffer from bloating, anxiety, and insomnia. Theirs is a windy, dry, and cool state, instead of a warm and moist Inner Climate®.

DOSHAS – The three functional forces that can define bio-individuality

	Qualities	Function	When in Excess
Kapha	Cold, dense, sluggish	Anabolic – growth	Over-nourished, heavy, and stagnant
Pitta	Hot and Moist	Metabolic – transformation	Hot and inflamed
Vata	Dry and Mobile	Catabolic – decline and movement	Dry and depleted

Doshic Balance is Warm and Moist

Ayurveda emphasizes that doshic balance is the main prerequisite for good health, and all Ayurvedic recommendations are designed to keep these three doshas doing their jobs in just the right ways. Even a slight imbalance in the doshas can create the potential for disease. But when kapha keeps growth at the right rate, pitta supports transformation and breakdown as needed, and vata allows things to move appropriately and to evacuate what's not needed, the body will be in perfect health.

Yet while all the Ayurvedic texts repeatedly state that "health is when these three doshas are balanced," and even describe what the body and mind might look like should they shift into imbalance, in the course of my research over the years I wasn't able to find a single statement that described what perfect balance actually looked like. Nevertheless, I refused to define perfect balance as just being about a lack of imbalance, or as health as simply being the lack of disease. There had to be a way of identifying what someone living in harmony at the perfect intersection of the three doshas would look like. And I had to find it, which I did, as I will shortly explain.

When things become overly hot and inflamed in the body, they can aggravate the pitta dosha. When unreasonably cool and sluggish, they aggravate kapha. But the midpoint of warmth keeps everything happy. When the body or mind becomes excessively dry, there is a vata imbalance; while the opposite, resulting in slime and accumulation, would be deemed as kapha aggravation. However, the midpoint of moist keeps all doshas doing their best.

To make it even more clear: When kapha's cool and fluid attributes become aggravated and excessive, the body tends to engage in excessive growth. In such cases, warmer and drier therapies are employed to restore a sense of warmth and moisture within the body, much like the summer sun melts the snow on our planet. It is essential to use these therapies judiciously, as overuse could potentially aggravate the heat of pitta and the dryness associated with vata, and dry us out like a hot desert.

In a similar manner, when the pitta dosha, characterized by its hot and humid qualities, becomes imbalanced, it requires the introduction of cool and dry elements in the appropriate measure to restore equilibrium. However, excessive cooling and drying therapies may contribute to an imbalance in the vata dosha instead, much like fall and winter affect the Earth. Likewise, when the dry and cool vata dosha is aggravated, this necessitates optimal warmth and moisture to maintain its well-being and restore balance.

Here's a handy table to sum up the qualities of each of the three doshas and how to address any imbalances.

Dosha	Qualities	When in excess, treat with:	Stop at the point when:
Kapha	cold and humid	warmth and dry	warm and moist
Pitta	hot and humid	cool and dry	warm and moist
Vata	cool and dry	warmth and moisture	warm and moist

Whenever I seek to balance a dosha, I treat it until it reaches a warm and moist state. Warm and moist is that sweet spot at which all three doshas are balanced, and the body and mind are in perfect health. It's when kapha isn't growing excess tissue or slime, pitta isn't heating and inflaming the system, and vata isn't acting like a destructive drying wind.

PRINCIPLE 2
THE CIRCADIAN RHYTHMS

As diurnal mammals, living according to six specific rhythmic cycles is essential for our healing and well-being.

To be completely honest with you, this principle was the basis for my family's daily routine when I was growing up and I learned it reflexively, almost like a first language. It was something that silently supported me in the way that oxygen does – and I took it equally for granted until about 12 years ago. Then, suddenly, I discovered an explosion of answers to unsolved problems, and I felt like Newton under that apple tree.

I now knew exactly why my client Lisa who worked late shifts as a waitress, was always bloated, even though her diet and exercise routines were impeccable. I understood why Missy kept gaining unhealthy weight, even though she exercised for a minimum of 60 minutes and consumed no more than 1500 Ayurvedic calories daily, out of which over 800 were ingested at dinner. And why Arun, a busy banker who loved his evening spin class, suffered from insomnia. I could even see why Angela's periods were still unpleasant and unpredictable after three months of taking herbs and treatments. It turned out that not following this second principle was a major reason behind most of the chronic imbalances I witnessed.

The Epiphany

I vividly remember the warm spring day in 2012 when I first felt the urge to revisit the principle of the circadian rhythms. My sister and I had just returned from the forests of Madhya Pradesh, North India, after what the rangers at the Pench National Park had called a "successful sighting day." Yet my personal sense of success came not only from spotting the wild creatures but from witnessing the keen sensitivity that all animals and birds displayed to the changes in their environment.

The morning safari had in fact probably been unremarkable for the rangers, but it was fascinating to me, as the silent dawn forest suddenly filled with the cries of birds, monkeys, deer, and chinkara (a type of gazelle); just a few minutes after sunrise, they arrived in a timely fashion to forage for their first meal of the day. Soon after, the mating calls of various animals merged to make music. However, the real adrenaline rush came from the warning sounds of birds and monkeys, signaling the presence of a predator nearby. These animals didn't use an organized language in the way that humans do, yet they could communicate not only with members of their own species but with other species as well. While my sister and I didn't glimpse a predator that morning, their sounds acted like an omen, persuading us to return for the evening safari, the ideal time to catch sight of a nocturnal hunter.

Sure enough, that evening, we drove back into the forest with the rangers over the uneven and muddy terrain, dust coating us and every surface of the vehicle. In the evolving darkness and amid increasingly loud warning cries, the silhouette of a leopard slowly emerged, its body draped over the branches of a teak tree. Its yellow-spotted torso was made dull by its blazing gaze as it looked around gracefully to scan its territory for food.

I froze before its beauty and its force, the darkness now illuminated only by dimmed Jeep headlights and bright leopard eyes. "Nocturnal nighttime vision," I remember repeating to myself silently, almost like a mantra, on the hour-long drive back, as I half listened to the rangers' stories of leopard kills and their subsequent midnight carcass feasts. The last time I'd comfortably digested a midnight feast was at the peak of my adolescence, in high school. Lucky leopards!

Back at our lodge, a couple hours after sunset, a beautiful bronze dinner plate filled with regional delicacies was set before me. There was a bowl of spiced lentils, perfectly crisp potatoes stained with turmeric, sautéed local greens, *roti* bread oozing with ghee, rice colored and flavored with saffron, peanuts, and red chilies mixed together in chutney, and plenty of other multicolored condiments that I couldn't name – but I can still recall the smell today; anyone could have confused such a meal with a carefully crafted sensory piece of art. But not me.

You see, I cannot help but examine everything in the world through my Ayurvedic lens – both my gift and my curse: "*As is the universe, such is the human body and vice versa*" is etched so deeply in my psyche that I constantly seek to make connections between the world outside myself and the world within me. So here were all six essential tastes (sweet, sour, salty, pungent, bitter, and astringent) perfectly combined and included in the meal in the manner that Ayurvedic wisdom recommends. But my thoughts kept returning to the words "nocturnal nighttime vision." Suddenly, the meal in front of me was no longer as appetizing. After all, we humans are diurnal beings, which means that we lack nighttime vision and at night our body essentially shuts down its daytime bodily functions, including digestion.

Before Thomas Edison bought bulbs to our homes, we followed the routines that nature meant for us to follow.

We allowed ourselves to be synchronized to the planet's clock, making it easier for the body to work, rest, and digest accordingly. Our ancestors practiced this wisdom as their natural way of life, not because of an expert's recommendation backed by scientific evidence.

And in case you're wondering, I did eat most of the delectable dinner on my plate, but not without mulling over it at the table, and discomfort later that night. Over the next few days, I revisited the principle in my thoughts and in the *Ashtanga Hrudayam Sutrasthana*, the most revered ancient Ayurvedic text, a bible for us doctors. I also perused modern medical research papers to understand the fluctuations in the brain and the corresponding chemical shifts in our body as the day progresses.

Each of the six Kalas – separate phases of a 24-hour period as described in Ayurveda – carries a distinct energy in the world outside and, therefore, in the world inside us. All life on the planet is aligned with the cycles of the sun and the moon, and depending on the phase of the day, the juices flowing in your body will vary in support of a specific function or activity. For example, melatonin, the sleep hormone, is produced when your eyes sense darkness, and insulin, a hormone that regulates blood sugar levels, gradually declines after sunset, making it harder for the body to break down late-evening starchy meals. "There's a time for everything" really holds true in this respect. Ayurvedic texts talked about this innate wisdom a few thousand years before the modern world rediscovered the power of the circadian rhythms and the human master clock, the suprachiasmatic nucleus (SCN), which is located in the brain.

What are the Circadian Rhythms?

The word *circa* means "about" in Latin, while *dian* comes from "day." Hence, the "circadian rhythms" are those natural cycles of physical, mental, and behavioral changes that happen in living things over the course of a 24-hour day. Light and darkness are the main influences that affect these rhythms, but other factors like eating, stress, exercise, social interactions, and temperature can also play a role. Thus, the second principle in this book is that all our internal functions will be enhanced and it will be easier for us to find and stay in balance when we dance to the tune of the circadian rhythms.

According to Ayurveda, day and night each have three separate sub-phases, adding up to a total of six distinct phases in a 24-hour period. The first three phases of the day are when the sun's energies are at their highest, and all things diurnal are in action mode. I call this the solar experience. The sub-phases of the solar experience are marked by the sun's rise, the sun's peak and the sun's decline. During this time, the wet Earth wakes up, becomes heated up, enabling its resources to be utilized for transformation, and eventually dehydrates from the power of the sun as evening arrives. A similar situation occurs in our bodies.

As the Earth shies away from the sun and turns to face the moonlight, we enter the lunar experience, supportive of repair. This comprises the onset of the night, the peak of the night, and the end of the night. During this time, the Earth cools down, gets ready to shut shop, falls into repair as deep darkness approaches, and then gradually awakens with replenished juices to prepare for a new dewy dawn – as does our body.

During the course of this chapter, I am going to teach you about the evolving phases of the 24-hour cycle and the unique opportunities that each one presents so you can optimize your well-being and find flow throughout the day. I ask not for blind faith, but for you to engage with the curiosity and alertness of those jungle creatures, ever in tune with their environment. That way, you will forge your own connections, discover personal truths and align your own rhythms.

When I talk about the phases, I'll touch upon some neuro-science, such as the neurotransmitters and hormones that come into force to support each of the specific phases. Some of these terms may be new to you; I invite you to look past the terminology and think of them as juices that facilitate changes in the brain and the body. Or you can choose to tune in and befriend them and make some notes if that helps. Studying these chemicals as precursors to changes in the body has become a new area of interest for modern science, and chances are that you'll hear a lot more about them in the coming years.

One more thing: The following breakdown assumes a 6am sunrise and 6pm sunset. However, depending on the season, the timing and length of certain phases can vary. If you feel more ambitious, feel free to tweak accordingly as you begin to practice this principle in Part 3. But even if you were to follow the existing breakdown, irrespective of your season or location, your body would experience a significant positive shift.

When we look at this from the lens of the Inner Climate®, the solar and lunar experiences perfectly align to ensure that the Earth experiences the "warm and moist" conditions necessary for life to thrive, and where the hot and dry aspects of the sun are balanced by the coolness and moisture facilitated by the moonlight. As we know, very little can grow and thrive without this optimum climate, as is the case in the cold extremities and dry deserts of the world, which have imbalanced or extreme solar and lunar experiences.

The Solar Experience	Heats and dries	Time for transformation and productivity	Doing	When balanced, perfect place of warm and moist
The Lunar Experience	Cools and moistens	Time for rest and repair	Being	

The Solar Experience

Imagine a bright sunny day; perhaps the very thought brings a smile to your face. The daytime hours are the optimum time for exercise and work, for eating and activity. In fact, the sun makes it possible for life to exist on Earth, so surely we can never get too much of it? But we all know that the sun can burn us and cause dehydration, thus requiring us to rest.

As a side note here, I want to introduce you to a novel concept. While our focus in this chapter is on the solar and lunar experiences brought about by the sun and moon, such experiences aren't limited to our exposure to these celestial bodies. Anything that has the power to dry and heat us can be considered solar, while anything that has the power to bring in moisture can be considered lunar.

The truth is that most of us have become too solar, drying out our essence through various means. Stress, anger, caffeine, alcohol, overly restrictive diets, insufficient sleep, excessive work and overtraining are just a few ways we subject ourselves to a "solar" lifestyle. These activities drain our vitality, leaving us parched and brittle like an autumn leaf, more like human doers than beings, and accelerating our wear and tear. While the rest of the book will address how you can move towards the center (neither too solar nor lunar) in all areas of your life, this chapter focuses on creating balance by utilizing the opportunities present during the actual phases of the day.

The Solar Experience – Phase I

The Fresh Morning Hours (6am to 10am)
The sun rises to gradually warm the Earth, which is still cool, wet, and dewy from the night. If you were to tune in to the sounds and activities of other diurnal species, you'd see that they are slowly beginning to pick up their pace now. The planet is still not fired up fully and, as diurnal beings, our

bodies witness a similar reality. After the lunar experience, humans wake up slightly cold, bodily fluids thicken, and mucus production is enhanced. The appearance of early morning nasal congestion and eye boogers is not uncommon for those who are prone to this. At the same time, synovial fluids thicken and create stiffness in the joints. No wonder morning yoga requires such a thorough warm-up and stretch routine before you can show off your flexibility. The gastric juices have been inactive for a while, rendering the Agni – the usually warm metabolic environment in the gut – slightly cold and soggy.

As our eyes begin to detect light, our level of serotonin – our feel-good hormone – begins to rise, giving us that hopeful feeling of a "new day." Drawing open the curtains to let that sunlight peek through will enhance our serotonin production. This is also when we experience rising levels of cortisol, a steroid hormone that regulates a wide range of vital processes throughout the body, including stress, metabolism, and the immune response; this allows sugar to enter the bloodstream and raise our energy so we can step into wakefulness. The dawn phenomenon, a condition where blood sugar levels elevate between the hours of 3am and 8am, is typical for most. This makes morning a great time to exercise, fire up the body and let it pick up pace. Exercise will naturally lower cortisol and start the regulation of blood sugar.

Exercise should ideally be followed by a quick shower and then breakfast. But a breakfast rich in fruits would be counterintuitive at this point. Yes, you read that right. Fruit is identical to the soggy, sugary, cold, and mushy environment of the body. In fact, the world's current morning fruit obsession would make my Ayurvedic grandfather grimace. If you were to study the diets of the blue zones, those places on Earth where people live exceptionally long lives, you would discover that they don't load their bodies with fruit early in the morning. I suspect the fruit-for-breakfast trend emerged as a better alternative to processed meats, Pop Tarts and sugary cereals. So yes, if cereals loaded with high-fructose corn syrup are your go-to, I can see why fruit would be deemed a healthier choice.

Rob, a client who was otherwise very compliant and easy to work with, wasn't yet ready to surrender his morning fruit smoothie. His post-nasal drip had become an inherent part of his being, until he was posted to a remote town in South America on a work project for three months. Here, making a morning smoothie wasn't easy, and in his words, "It was too tedious to bite into and chew fruit in the morning." *Voilà!* Within the first few weeks, his congestion began to clear and by the time he returned to NYC, the post-nasal trouble had been solved; his face was much less puffy and looked much brighter. And yes, neither his nasal drip nor the smoothies reappeared upon his return to NYC.

Ideally, the day's first meal should be a small and warm breakfast as an antidote to the barely fired-up gut, spiced in some manner to bring even more warmth. Complex carbohydrates like oatmeal, beans, whole grains, starchy veggies and lentils can support and stabilize blood sugar levels. My first meal for the day usually includes a handful of blanched and peeled almonds and a cup of hot, spiced, organic whole milk. And while my reason for consuming this combination is perfectly Ayurvedic, it's now established that dairy can enhance serotonin production and almonds contain magnesium, which lowers morning cortisol. Occasionally, I'll add some oatmeal to this mix. But I'll tell you more about this in Part 3, where I'll guide you through making these changes to your life one day at a time.

The Solar Experience – Phase II

The Hot Midday Hours (10am to 2pm)
As the sun picks up intensity, the heat and light on the planet increase on the side that is facing it, and the plants get ready for photosynthesis. Similarly, your body, which was gradually giving up its cold spell, is significantly warmer by now and

ready for the most productive part of the human day, which is between the hours of 10am and 2pm. The hormone norepinephrine peaks in this phase, bringing about what it is best known for: alertness and attention. Serotonin also reaches its maximum levels for the day, helping us to feel happy and inspired. No wonder these are usually the busiest, most productive and focused hours in schools and offices. This is the best time of day to use your analytical and rational mind.

But heat is not limited to the mind. As the sun peaks at midday, so does the fire in our belly. When people skip or delay lunch, it's not uncommon to see them get hangry (hungry plus angry), as all that fire needs food and fuel, or it can burn you up. Also, insulin has the potential to be most effective around then. A hormone produced by the pancreas, insulin is your body's answer to elevated blood sugar levels. A natural insulin peak supports the breakdown of sugars and complex starchy foods, making this a great time to consume the largest and most complex meal of the day – lunch.

I would recommend eating a freshly cooked, generous, and well-balanced lunch on most days that includes some complex carbohydrates, lentils or beans, good fats, greens, veggies, and spices. But this is also the time when you can live a little; your body's warm and juicy reality makes this the best time to indulge in all the foods you've been dreaming about. And if you haven't overdone your breakfast, ghrelin, the hunger hormone produced by the stomach, is probably on the rise, so this will also quieten down post-lunch. With regulated blood sugar, pacified ghrelin and insulin still in your system, your digestion is at the top of its game, your body is satiated and your chances of reaching for sugary, salty snacks or just any snacks are at their lowest. Why would anyone want to steer away from benefiting from these natural opportunities and rhythms?

The Solar Experience – Phase III

The Windy Early Evening Hours (2pm to 6pm)

The untimely daytime yawn, the body's unmistakable signal that we have hit the mid-afternoon phase. Right around 3.30 to 4pm, many of us find ourselves in the grip of an afternoon slump and reflexively lean back in our chair to stretch our arms and then probably wander over to the coffee machine. Well, we're not alone in this; most diurnal species and, in fact, even the planet itself can relate to it. Shortly after 2pm, the revolution of the Earth reduces its exposure to the sun's intensity on one side, and as the heavy, humid afternoon air evaporates, the wind begins to pick up. Yawning and the desire to stretch to drive out the wind trapped in our stationary joints are indicators of the subtle, rising breeze in our own bodies. After all, as is the macro, so is the micro. Almost all the juices, aka the hormones and neurotransmitters that support our most awake phase, including norepinephrine, cortisol and serotonin, start to decline. The body is beginning to shut down its resources for engagement and digestion. As insulin levels start to decline, so does the body's ability to break down complex carbohydrates and regulate blood sugar.

Our natural circadian rhythms intended us to honor the dimming daylight and subsequently dim down our own activities for the day, but electricity, innovation, and the desire for economic progress have demanded that we extend our working day and blur the line between the diurnal and the nocturnal. If your workday demands that you keep at your job after 4pm, I'd advise you to get a breath of fresh air if possible, stretch those limbs to allow the wind in your system to dissipate, enjoy a cup of peppermint or tulsi tea and a couple of sweet dates, splash some cool water on your face, and then return to your desk or work station. Reserve the easiest and most mindless tasks for this last bit of the solar phase. And if you have the luxury of calling it a day and stopping work, tune in to the mellowing sounds of the late afternoon, like birdsong if possible. Either way, gradually disconnect from the day and your phone, dim the lights, and play gentle evening music as you reach the tail-end of this phase at around 6pm.

The gut, too, experiences its own version of this unwinding wind, especially closer to the end of this phase. Colicky babies may find their bellies at maximum distention during these hours, and bloat is at its most extreme for all. Insulin production wants to step down rather than support the breakdown of blood sugar, and acetylcholine, the substance that stimulates the churning of gastric juices upon the smell or touch of food, is at its lowest point in its natural circadian cycle.

We are meant to be supper beings rather than dinner beings. Indeed, a few centuries ago, before electricity illuminated our homes, dining was a far simpler affair, a world away from the elaborate dinner spreads adorned with multiple dishes that we might imagine today. Our ancestors, guided by the rhythms of the sun and the limitations of daylight, leaned toward more practical and sustainable cooking methods. They consumed hearty, fat-rich broths and stews, slowly simmered over open fires in robust stone pots. This cooking method not only maximized the natural flavors and nutrients of the ingredients but also introduced the concept of "eating" your soup, a nourishing, all-encompassing meal crafted from the simplicity and necessity of their times. Although human bodies are constantly adapting and evolving to newer lifestyles and dietary choices, it will take a few million years before our gut learns how to digest and break down dinner effectively.

After this last of the three phases that complete the solar experience, activity on the planet and inside our bodies quietens, and a world of healing and repair emerges.

The Lunar Experience

Before diving into the lunar experience, I must emphasize its importance – a theme you'll notice both in this chapter and throughout the book. To counteract the effects of our shift toward the solar experience, we need to infuse our lives with the nourishing aspects of the moon. Embracing the lunar experience by honoring the cycles of this second phase can offer a prime chance to achieve equilibrium. However, the lunar experience is not limited to the lunar hours. It can also be brought in through meditation, breathwork, practicing gratitude and compassion, mindful eating, incorporation of healthy fats in our diet, and listening to classical music, for example, among other strategies that enhance our rest and nourishment, something which I will detail further in the book.

The Lunar Experience – Phase I

The Unwinding Night Hours (6pm to 10pm)
This phase marks the dramatic shift from day to night, as the sun sets, birds return to their roosts and diurnal animals retire to their hiding places, mindful of nocturnal predators.

When I was a young teen, I liked to stay out in the park with my friends way past dusk. After several late returns and gentle reprimands, my mother made a compromise, telling me, "Come home when you see bats weaving through the sky." Somehow, this advice resonated deeply with me, transcending the ordinary limits of parental authority. It was nature's own cue to slow down and settle down, and so I surrendered.

The body experiences a significant transition during this period; the daytime excitatory substances that kept our nervous system engaged and supported our physical endeavors during the solar experience now naturally start dialing back. As darkness hits the eyes, serotonin, the "feel good neurotransmitter" known for mood regulation and anxiety, is converted to the "sleep hormone," melatonin.

This also explains why some people may feel a sudden bout of anxiety at dusk.

At the same time, adenosine, which builds up during the daytime, increases sleep pressure, and gamma-aminobutyric acid (GABA), the "calming neurotransmitter," seems to be more active now. Basically, your body wants you to unwind. Yes, we can create a simulated bright, active, noisy day-like environment and confuse our master clock – the suprachiasmatic nucleus (SCN) located in the hypothalamus – that it's daytime. However, I'm not convinced that it's a good idea to go against the tide and regularly violate the hypothalamus's natural rhythms. After all, the hypothalamus is the master endocrine gland that controls the release of almost all of the body's hormones and neurotransmitters, which are now known to play a significant role in many autoimmune conditions.

Rather, I'd recommend a nighttime ritual to celebrate the lunar phase and to prepare the body for rest. Turning down the dimmer switch of your artificial lighting and everything else that keeps you excited and awake is a great way to enter this phase. You can use soft music and natural floral aromas to enhance this experience further.

You've probably already heard repeatedly about the importance of keeping away from screens during this phase, but I'm still going to say it again. The blue light given out by a screen won't allow all that lovely serotonin to convert to your sleep-time juice, melatonin. The screen confuses the brain and unsettles the nervous system, and there is no signaling for rest and, in fact, there may even be a build-up of anxiety instead. However, journaling does the opposite. It allows you to process and assimilate what's happened in the day, integrates and grounds the nervous system, and sets you up for slumber so you can be "melatoning" by 10pm.

This phase is ideally a food-free phase. However, the earliest part of this phase, i.e. 6pm, is typically when a light dinner or supper can be enjoyed.

The Lunar Experience – Phase II

The Repair Night Hours (10pm to 2am)

The word "repair" falls short when it comes to conveying the full power of this period. As the night darkens and the planet settles down after sunset, an active healing and recovery phase begins, all while you are cozy and comfortable in your bed. We, as humans, couldn't have asked for a better bargain. While the body is in a seemingly effortless place, inside, your neurotransmitters, cells, and the glymphatic system, which clears waste out of your central nervous system, are working hard so you can process, eliminate, and repair anything in the body that causes a lack of equilibrium. The caveat is that the conscious mind should be asleep so deep work can happen within.

Let's take a look at what happens. As most of the excitatory mediators of the brain slow down their activity, the impact of GABA, the calming neurotransmitter, increases and enables serotonin to be converted to melatonin, the sleep hormone, so a state of slumber can be gradually induced. However, if there is a significant exposure to blue light, this chemical shut-down doesn't happen effectively.

If you do fall into deep sleep, growth hormone – which plays a key role in body composition, cell repair, and metabolism – has its strongest surge. Growth hormone is joined by prolactin, which also effects the immune system and metabolism, so the body can enjoy repair at the most microscopic level. Not only that, but did you know that thinking creates debris in the nervous system? No wonder we modern-day intellectual beings face a host of mental disorders and challenges. Well, deep sleep allows your glymphatic system to become active. While researchers are still exploring this system, we know that it facilitates the clearance of mental waste from the central nervous system (CNS) and operates more efficiently during sleep, thanks to the changes in the brain's environment that occur during this time. Long story short, make sure that you can take advantage of the repair phase and get as much sleep as possible in these hours.

Now, if you have decided that you're a night owl rather than a lark, know that this is merely your preference and that your biological self is unfamiliar with the concept; I doubt that 300 years ago our ancestors lit a lamp and hung around outside their homes, star-gazing in the middle of the night, just because they believed they were nocturnal. In fact, when you stay up until the wee hours, your body consumes twice the amount of energy as it does during the day, as it's trying to run all its systems at once, but none effectively.

If your body tries to play this awake but sleepy game, it heats up; think of a car that has driven more miles than the engine can handle. With all this heat in the system, it's not uncommon for a person to feel hungry. You can pacify this urge with a warm cup of whole milk, spiced with cardamom or nutmeg, right before bedtime. If you give into that hunger pang with anything more substantial, your already taxed system has an added task of digestion without the resources that it requires to achieve this. Over a period of time, such a lifestyle can lead to severe imbalances and even chronic disease.

When Adam, a financial advisor from NYC, filled out his near-impeccable food and lifestyle journal prior to meeting with me, I remember thinking to myself, "What on Earth could have led to the recent onset of severe constipation and dryness that were listed as his top goal for working with me?" I was surprised by how depleted he looked when he walked in – his eyes sullen, with dark crescents under them, his skin parched, and his gait weary. I remember thinking that he had probably experienced some serious tragedy and there, I felt, lay the answer.

But upon investigation, I discovered that, in fact, no such thing had occurred, but instead he'd developed a serious addiction to the video games on his phone in recent months. He confessed to staying up late every single night, occasionally into the small hours of the morning. It took some convincing before he would finally believe that his slow bowel movements and dryness had any connection to his sleep. Being the conscientious person he was, once convinced, he went all out to incorporate lunar elements into his life, most importantly, getting his timely sleep. Within the span of four to five weeks, he emailed me, saying, "Out of the video games and back in the game :-). Thank you!" And I haven't heard from him since.

The Lunar Experience – Phase III

The Dead of the Night Hours (2am to 6am)
The first part of this period (2am to 4am) is the deep night, probably the most inactive period for the majority of species on the planet. The diurnal and crepuscular creatures (those active at dawn and dusk) are resting and the nocturnal have completed their primary period of activity. During this silent time in the 24-hour period, the body has completed most of its internal repair work. Depending on the Inner Climate® of an individual, we may wake up at this hour to urinate or, perhaps, in a sweat. Growth hormone is still at its peak and post-repair rebuilding continues. However, the nervous system begins to free up after all that thought-debris has been processed by the glymphatic system. The body moves now into longer periods of REM sleep or light sleep, making it harder to fall asleep if awoken, especially the closer we get to 4am. With the newly created space in the nervous system, it becomes easy for us to become anxious or experience racing thoughts if awake during this phase. My recommendation would be to stay asleep during these hours if you can. However, if not, keep your eyes closed and resist the temptation to check the time or switch on your screen. Stay away from light as much as you can, so you can align with the natural circadian rhythms. Yoga nidra, a deep relaxation technique, can be very useful to maintain a rest state, even if the body wakes.

In Part 3, I will offer some suggestions for maximizing the benefits of this lunar phase.

Shortly after 4am, the rooster crows and we shift into even lighter sleep – not from the sound of crowing but from the gradual activation of daytime excitatory mediators in the body, like norepinephrine and acetylcholine; the latter gets your heart and intestinal peristalsis pumping. With a little support from its rising serotonin levels, your body is now preparing for a timely bowel movement. Timely, according to the Ayurvedic circadian rhythm, means shortly after sunrise. After all, its waste matter has been processed in the repair phase, and your body wants a fresh start. It is not uncommon for members of traditional Ayurvedic households in India to attempt bowel evacuation immediately upon waking. Chances are that this isn't the case for you. Unfortunately, I've heard modern-day doctors consider it normal for a patient to have a bowel movement once every few days. But the principle is simple: You eat every day, you go every day.

When Yana came to me, she was working simultaneously with two other Ayurvedic doctors, who had put her on a long list of herbs. Already following an Ayurvedic diet, she had found relief from several of her symptoms, but her constipation and inflammation markers for rheumatoid arthritis remained unchanged. I refused to add any more herbs to the list and, in fact, strongly suggested that she minimize her herbal intake. I also had no doubt that her inflammation was linked to her constipation. The backlog of undigested, stuck food in a warm-blooded body can only lead to fermentation inside, which in turn can cause inflammation. I slightly altered her diet, but more than anything, I worked with her to honor the natural rhythms of the sun and the moon.

Within three weeks, she was having a proper bowel movement every day, and that too, in the morning. On her next blood exam, her inflammation markers had greatly reduced and she was now down from taking over a dozen herbs to just a couple. Yana's story offers hope to the constipated population of the world. Once you align with the order of the universe and eat and live in a way that optimizes your Inner Climate®, it is only a matter of time until a squat on the pot becomes a daily morning activity.

Traditionally, yogis and the spiritually seeking woke up shortly after 4am for meditation to take advantage of theta brain waves in these wee hours of the morning. During this phase, called the *Brahma Mahurta*, brain wave frequencies are associated with enhanced creativity, memory consolidation, emotional processing, increased intuition, and even reduced anxiety. Ever since he was a young boy, my grandfather used to rise early to use this opportunity to regulate and explore his inner world. Inspired by his example, I chose to study in the hours of the early morning, as opposed to burning the midnight oil like my peers did in high school.

So, if you find yourself awake after 4am, I would strongly recommend staying away from your phone and remaining in your lunar experience by using this time to meditate, introspect, write, chant or learn something new. But if you don't have an agenda like that, it's preferable to stay asleep and allow your body to wake up naturally with the sunrise, but not later. Sleeping way past sunrise will inevitably make the body sluggish and means that it will miss the opportunity for natural peristalsis. After all, the next phase, between 6am and 10am, is when the body is naturally in a soggy state, and sleeping beyond this point can tip you into a state of lunar imbalance. Hence the earlier recommendation to get moving and warm up between the 6am to 10am solar phase.

Tune in to the Solar and Lunar Phases

Now, since you know about the six phases of the day, my ask is that you begin to tune in to the energies outside and within you. Can you feel the sluggishness in the morning, the heat building up with the rising sun, and can you tune in to the dry wind in the early evening? Here's a table to help you get started.

TIME	PREDOMINANT ENERGIES	ACTIVITY	FOOD
6am to 10am	Wet and sluggish	Warm up, exercise, get moving	Warm breakfast and warm beverage
10am to 2pm	Hot and metabolic	Focus on everyday tasks	Biggest meal (lunch)
2pm to 6pm	Windy and depleting	Wind down slowly	3.30pm peppermint tea
6pm to 10pm	Earth and grounding	Connect and introspect	6pm – small dinner 9.30pm – hot milk
10pm to 2am	Silent internal repair	Sleep	Sleep
2am to 6am	Etheric and subtle	Sleep or meditate	Sleep

Look at the world around you and make connections. I have been doing this mindfully for over a decade, and subconsciously for a lifetime. Yet I still find new associations and fresh reasons for awe each and every single day.

However, if your tendency is to take new information and put protocols in place instantly, narrowing the scope of your flow in the name of a healthy life, let me ask you to take a moment and draw in some lunar energy instead of letting the burden of a so-called healthy lifestyle burn you out before you really begin. Internalize these rhythms through keen observation and, for now, only make those changes that feel natural and effortless to you. In Part 3, I will show how you can align yourself with your circadian rhythms and apply the three principles to all the core areas of your life.

PRINCIPLE 3
GROWTH, TRANSFORMATION, AND DECLINE

Growth, transformation, and decline are the three inevitable phases of all cycles.

"Death is certain for one who has been born, and rebirth is inevitable for one who has died" – this particular verse from the *Bhagavad Gita*, a Vedic scripture full of life lessons weaved into an epic poem, emphasizes the transience of life and yet offers hope of another chance for rebirth: While this particular statement refers to human life, it also sits at the core of Principle 3. Life does itself in three phases: growth, transformation, and decline. These phases exist everywhere, from the smallest cell to the largest organism, to the largest organization. They apply too to the phases of the day and the seasons, to our relationships and even our lifecycle, as well as to the intangible aspects of life.

Each year, *growth* on Earth starts increasing with the wetness of spring, warms and *transforms* into summer, and then dries and *declines* in fall (or autumn) and the winter months. If you were to step foot on the planet for the first time on a bitter winter's day and didn't know better, you might think our planet is always covered in dead vegetation. But instead you know that these are phases; the winter will meet spring again, and thus, you can embrace the cold, lifeless months in the hope of new life. This cyclical reality isn't limited to the seasons; it applies to everything, the micro and the macro, from every single cell in the body to the body as a whole and beyond to all things on the planet.

But what does this principle have to do with us living a healthier and happier life? Firstly, it allows us to zoom out and appreciate the transience of everything while offering hope for the new. The phase of decay is always followed by a new phase of growth. This invites surrender and allows us to stay in flow. Even if you aren't the "this too shall pass" type, this principle allows you to understand the world around you better and thus naturally become more mindful of your relationship with everything.

The good news is that you probably already do this unknowingly in many instances. For example, imagine that you're growing some mangoes in your backyard, and the fruit on the tree isn't ready to eat yet; you'd inherently know that it's in the *growing* phase and probably needs more nurturing, water and sunlight before it matures for consumption. This feels like a natural, intuitive choice rather than an expert-led decision. After waiting for it to *transform* into its ripe and juicy form, you deem that it's fit to enjoy. But if you miss this phase, the fruit will start to *decay* and then you will have to wait for another season so the cycle can repeat itself.

Now, this quality of mindful interaction is easier with the mango because its growth cycle is evident, and most of us have had first-hand experience with something like it. But sometimes, we will need to look deeper to understand the current phase of an entity's lifecycle so we can make more intuitive, effortless choices that will enhance our well-being and flow. My job here is to teach you how to magnify and deepen your lens so you can make that happen.

The Growth Phase

The growth phase is usually characterized by increase in size and bulking up, made possible by rapid cell proliferation. And since 70 to 90 percent of any cell mass is typically made of water, fluid elements are almost always involved in this phase. Additionally, when anything is in the growth phase, heat is mild and only gradually builds up so it can eventually move into the productive transformation phase. The prerequisites to getting the growth phase right are the right amount of fluid raw materials and appropriate amounts of gradual heat. Basically, we're back to our old friends warm and moist, but things tend to get a little more moist compared to warm in this phase, and maintaining a delicate balance between the two is essential for balance.

Let's use the analogy of a seed here. When the seed is planted in the wet soil, the growth phase begins. It needs frequent watering during this phase till it develops its own roots and is able to draw up water from the ground. With the right amount of irrigation and moderate sunlight, roots grow and the seed erupts into a sapling. Too much water will cause fungi, clogging, and improper growth. Too much sunlight will dry the moisture and the sapling will wither. Now, if things go right, the sapling will successfully move into the transformation phase, where the real blossoming happens. The need for frequent watering diminishes at this point.

To support any growth phase, it's important to provide the right raw materials and conditions for growth, but at the same time, to induce heat strategies slowly so stagnation doesn't occur. Let me make it even clearer.

The morning can be considered as the growth phase of the day. Things are still wet and are moving toward the ripe, most productive part of the day. If you stayed in bed late and consumed cold, dense smoothies in the morning instead of supporting the growing heat, you would feel even more sluggish. No wonder oversleeping doesn't bring rest; it brings lethargy. It doesn't allow you to be active and productive during the day. As we've seen, the antidote is to wake up at an appropriate time, fire things up through exercise, and eat a small, warm breakfast.

Similarly, childhood is the growth phase of human life; our bodies and minds are more fluid, our tissues grow rapidly, and the heat of adolescent hormones is gradually building. Childhood is thus the perfect time to build a foundation for learning, memories, immunity, and all else. Even though we cannot see it, the body supports the churning of fluid elements for raw materials like cytoplasm, the gel-like substance that makes up the bulk of a cell. Along with it comes the side effect of quick and rapid phlegm at the smallest deviation, making children more prone to runny colds than adults. When supported with the right foods, the body knows how to build not only new cells but also protective lymph that will support immunity, soft mucosal lining in the gut that will support the microbiome, and the gel-like myelin sheath that will keep nerves functioning well. Notice how the cytoplasm, lymph, mucosal lining, and myelin sheath have similar fluid textures.

When I had my second child Sanjali, my four-year-old firstborn Suhani had just started preschool. She was a bright, healthy girl who had been raised so far according to the three principles described in this book. With only slight trepidation, I was ready to let her into the wild world. But soon, she developed a peculiar and recurrent fever pattern. Every three weeks, she would get sick, and her temperature would shoot up to 102.5°F (39°C). Previously energetic and rarely unwell, she would now become easily and seriously congested, lethargic and dull. I would inevitably step in with my fever protocols, and somehow, on the second night, her fever would naturally break sometime between 10pm and 2am. This went on for about four months.

Preoccupied with the new baby, I outsourced the investigation to her pediatrician, who found no concrete answers. Eventually, we were referred to a rheumatologist and gastroenterologist for further testing. The latter ordered instructions for an endoscopy and colonoscopy, for which Su would have to fast for a few hours, drink copious amounts of a colored liquid, and cameras would be inserted into her tender gullet and other body orifices.

By this stage, I'd had enough and I declined the testing. I decided to put on my Ayurvedic hat and take things into my own hands. I knew that Su was in her growth phase of life and therefore vulnerable to phlegm and stagnation. Upon investigation, I discovered that she had developed a fondness for the cold banana milkshake at her new preschool and often consumed multiple servings. The preschool assistants were also overfeeding her, and as a four-year-old, Su's gut lacked the fire necessary to break down large amounts of food effectively. Both factors were the raw materials of the very worst kind, especially for this stage of her development – sticky, cold, and humid.

I changed around a few things, eliminated the milkshake, and added warm and moist foods such as rice congee with ginger powder, spiced lentils or rice, warm milk with turmeric, and the occasional neti pot (a form of nasal irrigation). *Voilà!* Suhani's peculiar fever never returned.

Millions of children whose parents never make this connection suffer, and I'm not surprised to see the growing rate of allergies, asthma, and even juvenile diabetes. Similarly, there's a reason why spring, the growth time of the planet, brings with it severe allergies. This is also the reason why excess rain in the spring causes waterlogging and fungal diseases.

If you like the language of the doshas, the growth phase is essentially a kapha phase.

To summarize, this phase naturally pushes the Inner Climate® to be slightly more humid and brings with it a vulnerability to stagnation. It can be supported by the gradual introduction of moderate heat so things keep moving forward in their lifecycle. (I will address more protocols for these growth phases in Part 4.)

The Transformation Phase

The second phase represents the pinnacle of productivity within the lifecycle. It's during this stage that any form of life finds that its purpose and its contribution to the planet is fulfilled the most. This is when fruits ripen and are ready to eat; when humans arrive at adolescence and are able to procreate and use all the knowledge they've built up before this in the workforce; and this is when the mitochondria, the powerhouse of the cell, gets to work on generating the chemical energy needed for the cell's biochemical reactions. This is the phase every modern-day scientist wants to hack. How do we keep our youth forever? And how might we preserve a fruit in its ripe state for longer or lengthen the life of mitochondria? How can we stay productive for more hours?

If you examine this phase, you will notice a few things. Transformation occurs when the growing phase peaks, usually marked by an entity reaching its full size. Secondly, once that growth has been completed, it is heat that propels and tips things over into this phase. The growing phase is fluid-dominant, but this phase is heat-dominant. The warm sun ripens the fruit that has attained its full size; the hot hormones allow the full-grown child to experience puberty (hence, the passionate, hot-tempered teenager); the mitochondria get heated up for energy production, and daytime is the hottest part of the 24-hour period.

This phase starts out deviating from the warm and moist to "hot and moist" before it starts drying up as it approaches its end. Think of the face of the average 16-year-old girl with oily skin, perhaps with some fluid-filled acne spots, and bubbling with hormones; in other words, with "hot and moist" written all over it. Yet by the time most women are in their thirties, they often begin to complain of some sort of dryness. The fruit that was ripe and juicy at the start of this transformation phase will eventually dry out and decay if left unused.

Another analogy I like to use is that of an oil lamp filled with fuel to the brim. You know that it has a long way to go before it loses its flame. But as time progresses, the fuel starts drying up, and eventually, the flame is extinguished. Similarly, in our own bodies, puberty starts out like that oil-filled lamp, and by the time we are in our late teens and twenties, not only are we often very fertile, but we are also at our most passionate and productive, both at work and otherwise.

Those who haven't abused their bodies will also have more forgiving digestive systems that demand bigger and more varied portions, but can handle these without developing any symptoms. After all, it's hot in there. But as we continue to burn our fuel, either through the natural course of time or due to our extremely solar lifestyles, we start to deplete the fuel supply and arrive at the tail end of the transformation cycle. Just like the charred end of a matchstick, the flame can no longer be fed and burns out. The secret to navigating this phase well is to preserve your fuel and use your fire wisely; to make sure that all your solar activities are being balanced by lunar antidotes; that work is balanced by rest, and that doing is balanced by being. Both are equally important: the fire and the fuel that sustains the fire.

I learned Adrienne's story on the day she joined me in a slow-flow yoga session, rather than turning left for her usual hot yoga class. Even though I hadn't spoken to her before, I had often seen her at the yoga studio. Her wrinkled skin and grey hair suggested that she was probably in her fifties, but she was on top of her yoga game, and today I had the opportunity to witness her skill as I practiced beside her. I was impressed with her headstand, her wheel pose, and her ability to hold the postures longer than anyone else. She wore protective knee and elbow pads. My curiosity got the better of me, and I struck up a conversation with her at the end of the class.

She was, in fact, only 46 and an ex-lawyer from Harvard. The long work hours, late nights, caffeine, and the intensity... She explained she couldn't take it anymore and had recently given up her legal practice to pursue her life-long love of the culinary arts. At the peak of her burnout, yoga was recommended to her, and she signed up for hot yoga right away. But recently, her joints had begun to crack and even feel inflamed, so her chiropractor suggested she slow down a little more, thus the slow-flow yoga. She was a classic example of premature fuel depletion, aka burnout. The dryness on her skin was visible, and once I knew her story, I could smell the smoke from her burnout. Unfortunately, due to a lack of proper guidance, she couldn't understand what was happening in her body and mind, and even when she sought recovery, she took to hot yoga, which only added to her heat and dryness.

Over a period of time, we became good friends, and she grew interested in my work. Today, Adrienne practices abhyanga (Ayurvedic self-massage), goes on long walks on moonlit nights, sleeps with water sounds, drinks less caffeine, practices yin yoga and generally looks much happier. Had she understood the changes that the body experiences through the three cycles, her burnout could have been potentially avoided.

Her story is quite different from Donia's. I worked with Donia, a 32-year-old Egyptian woman who was struggling to conceive. Her obesity was a result of over-nourishment in childhood and the excess consumption of stagnant foods like cheese, cold dairy products, and sugar. And even though menarche came quite early for her, as she started menstruating at the age of 11, her periods had been deeply painful, often heavy or blocked and irregular. Donia's body had become sluggish in childhood, and her transformation fire never kicked off fully; 20 years later, she was still suffering. She experienced inertia and lacked the passion to get out of bed most days. She had had a difficult childhood and was unable to process some of her experiences. After all, you need heat in your nervous system to transform memories into learnings and to move on.

The therapies that I suggested to Donia looked drastically different to those of Adrienne. Donia had never let the solar fully kick in, in a way that would allow her to enjoy the peak of the transformation phase. I'm glad she came to me in her early thirties so I could help her activate her latent fire, which would be a greater challenge as she would naturally move into the next phase. Her keywords became "stimulate, move, warmth, spice-up, passion." Even though her inherent nature was to retreat into inactivity, she was now warmed up. She became pregnant eight months later but was diagnosed with gestational diabetes, a condition of high blood sugar associated with pregnancy, which, to me, was no surprise.

For those Ayurvedic jargon lovers among you, this is the pitta phase in the lifecycle of an entity. It starts out bubbling and hot, like pitta, but it's vulnerable to premature burnout if the fuel isn't used mindfully and replenished. The body's Inner Climate® gets naturally pushed to become hotter. However, if there is inactivity and overconsumption, the flame will be too weak for the fuel and the result is stagnation. Alternatively, if the flame burns too fiercely, it will result in a quick burnout.

The Decline or Decay Phase

This marks the end of the productive phase and the start of a journey toward death, also known as aging, or the vata phase of life in Ayurveda. As morbid as it sounds, this is the reality for all life on the planet. And it is indeed the process that keeps our planet fresh, new, and evolving. Just as aged, degenerated cells would create an imbalance if they found permanent residence in your body, the Earth has a cleansing mechanism for all on the other side of their biologically productive phase, so space for the new can be created. I have learned that reverence for death as a result of aging is reverence for life, new life.

In practical terms, when the ripening and reproduction phases are complete, the process of aging starts. This is when the oil-filled lamp loses its fuel and thus its flame. The length of the three phases can greatly vary depending on the species, and there are certain creatures on the planet that experience negligible senescence or decline. But for our purposes, let's stick to our bodies and the everyday world we interact with.

The process of decline, as it occurs in its natural cycle, is almost always associated with a loss of water or dryness. Given that the building phase is water-dominant, then it's only natural for this phase to be the opposite – that is, drier. I often joke that we start out as grapes in our adolescence but end up as raisins when we age, the classic example of shrinkage due to fluid depletion. When all the oil from the lamp is used up, the flame shrinks and dry smoke emerges. Decay and decline are always marked by the loss of the ability to reproduce and the loss of the juice of life, as well as of transformative heat. The result is a drier, cooler phase that facilitates shrinkage, just like the autumn wind is the precursor to the leaves withering and falling off the trees.

For women, early signs of this phase start in their late thirties and early forties. Doctors often talk about pregnancies differently after the age of 35, calling them "high risk." That's because from about 35 to 45, things start to slow down. At this point, you might start noticing some changes – like your skin feeling drier, more wrinkles appearing, or your joints making more noise. These are little signs that things are starting to dry out a bit, kind of like when the wind blows and makes everything feel a bit parched.

As time goes on and menopause approaches, things change even more. Your body's natural juices, like those that keep your skin soft and your body feeling good, start to diminish. This can lead to things like dryness "down there," fewer natural oils in your skin, more wrinkles, and even a slower metabolism. You might have heard of hot flashes, too – those sudden feelings of heat that can come out of nowhere. They often show up during what's called perimenopause, right before menopause really kicks in. It's like your body's last hurrah before things start to wind down. If you are in this phase, you might even notice you're not as tall as you used to be: That's because the gel-like stuff in the discs of your spine starts to dry out, making you lose a bit of height. This phase naturally pushes the ideal warm and moist Inner Climate® to cool and dry.

But I'm here to guide, not to frighten. Understanding the aging process can help you to keep your inner flame burning while making the most of your fuel. In the tales shared earlier, Adrienne burned through her fuel too fast, leading to exhaustion, while Donia's fire lacked spark, leaving her feeling sluggish. In the modern urban world, I see more Adriennes rather than Donias. Imbalances that arise out of a lifestyle that's too solar will lead to burnout or inflammation, akin to global warming but inside the body. Either way, throughout this book, I'll be teaching you how to reconcile yourself with each of these phases in your own body, as well as how to identify them in the world around you, so you can make choices that enhance your outer and inner glow.

That being said, I can assure you that each one of us will still decay and meet our demise sooner or later. It's as sure as the fact that the evening will be followed by night, and autumn or fall will be followed by winter. But then our decayed bodies may mix with the soil and support more life, in the same way that the night will end in the morning and the winter will meet spring again. And when you respect these natural cycles as the inevitable seasons of life and time, you'll find more health, joy, and fulfillment.

Living in Harmony with the Three Phases

What makes these cycles even more interesting is that they aren't just limited to the physical and temporal aspects of our being and of the world around us, but can be extended to everything life touches.

To give you an example, if we were to consider a romantic relationship, the initial stage is usually about growth. You try to build a bond by spending time with your new love interest, being genuinely curious to learn and understand who they are – very juicy indeed! This phase is critical and often determines where the relationship will go next. If enough fire builds up, it can proceed to the transformation phase, where you and your loved one may decide to make things official. Then, as per the third principle, natural progression should see the relationship fall into a decline, but that doesn't have to be the case in this instance. Fortunately, when it comes to anything that isn't bound by the limitations of matter, the cycle has the ability to repeat and retain itself. In a partnership, if you continue to build on the backend, the relationship will continue to transform and reach new heights. If not, then decline is inevitable.

The same is true for our careers. We may get into a career of our choice, all gung-ho, acquiring the right education, and building a skillset so we can be productive and prove ourselves at the workplace. But once at work, if we don't keep growing and building, we can easily fall into decline in this dynamic, competitive world. In the same way, the largest organizations fail when they don't continue to build and innovate.

In the total realm of existence, one domain remains unaffected by the mundane laws of growth and decline, and that is the journey of spiritual awakening. As we explore the depths of our own being, seeking self-understanding and healing, we embark on a path of infinite growth and transformation. Here, there's no such thing as decline.

Instead, we find ourselves slowly shedding the layers of our ego, moving toward dissolution rather than decline. This quest, as ancient as the stars themselves, is in fact the most fulfilling adventure we can undertake, especially as we move beyond the vigor of youth. Even though this is a topic of its own, I wanted to plant a seed in your consciousness that you may continue to water, as the idea of transience in all other areas becomes evident.

PART 2
LIVING AYURVEDA

This is where the fun really begins. Now that Part 1 has taught you the principles, Part 2 will teach you to apply them to the main areas of your life.

People often tell me that understanding the three principles feels like putting on a new pair of glasses that give you super-vision, and you can never see yourself or the world in the same way again. To use another metaphor, they can become your power tool for cutting through all the marketing clutter in the wellness world, ensuring that you only adopt what passes the test of these principles. You can also think of the principles like three formulae that you can use to unlock pretty much any problem area in your life. This may sound far-fetched as of now, but as with any formula, it's practice that makes perfect. You want to start with the basic areas and eventually extend their application to other areas of your life so you can continue to unlock, heal, and grow.

As a recap, the three core principles are:

- **Principle 1. The Inner Climate®**: This refers to your inner state, which should ideally be warm and moist.

- **Principle 2. The circadian rhythms**: These are the natural cycles of the day, which can be divided into the solar and lunar experiences, which have three phases each.

- **Principle 3. Growth, transformation, and decline**: These are the three phases of every cycle, moving from moist to heat to dry, and from growth to transformation and decline.

We're now going to look at how to apply these principles to daily life. Take the following questions: *When and how do I exercise? What and when do I eat? How are the mind and body connected? How do I navigate through changing seasons?* We will answer all of these and more through the lens of the three principles. However, the ultimate goal of this section is not just to answer questions like these, but for you to learn to apply these codes to your own life. If you internalize this process, you can eventually start applying it to every single area of life, way beyond the ones covered in this book, as was the case for my client Mahika.

Mahika initially came to me for help with her gut and skin, but stayed on to learn about the three principles in more detail. A 33-year-old woman from Atlanta, Mahika had landed in a toxic relationship. As she started healing, she realized that love wasn't just a matter of checking boxes on her list, or the adrenaline rush, or even the desperate calling of her confused heart. She learned instead that she needed to find a long-term partner who would make her feel consistently warm and moist inside, and thus safe.

I'm going to call it out before you do. When I say "warm and moist" here, I mean the sweet gooeyness of love inside, but it isn't a coincidence that these terms are used to describe bodily fluids during a strong physical attraction to someone, preceding the actual act of the creation of life. After all, life can only thrive in a warm and moist place.

Mahika basically used the principle of the Inner Climate® to identify red flags and toxic interactions that made her feel hot, dry, and aggravated in her chest. She was able to release herself from her current relationship so she could restore balance and then invite a partner into her life who would feel like a cozy blanket rather than taking her on an emotional rollercoaster.

In contrast, I wasn't keen to work with Lasha initially; she only wanted a prescriptive diet plan to lose 20lb (9kg) for her sister-in-law's wedding. I set forth my conditions: I would only work with her if she were willing to understand how her body functions and then let weight-loss happen mainly as the side effect of healing. (She later disclosed that even though she was surprised by my request, she still agreed to work with me because I'd helped her cousin lose 40lb (18kg) without him having to give up carbs. To be honest, I'm still unsure whether the hook that wheeled her in was the 40lb or the carbs.)

Well, Lasha was a bright woman, and once she began to shake off her initial inertia, her world opened up. She understood intuitively that her stagnant Inner Climate® set her body on a constant growth phase, making transformation difficult for her. Eating processed cheese, sugar, and late dinners further exacerbated the problem. She also realized why she constantly felt stuck. Wearing her new three-principle glasses, it became effortless for her to move, stimulate herself, eat warmer foods, and feel better overall. At some point in our six months' consultancy together, she forgot all about her weight loss; instead, she simply embarked on a mission to restore balance in her Inner Climate® and live by the planet's rhythms. With this new warmth, she even rekindled some stuck, silent relationships. At the end of our time working together, she was 17lb (7.5kg) lighter, more radiant, visibly happier, slept much better, and was prepared to give up her data analytics job to teach art.

These two stories demonstrate the unlimited potential of the principles. But for now, I'd like you to focus on their application in your own life and then to internalize whatever resonates with you. If you feel called to do so now, simply implement those changes that feel the most natural and require the least effort. At this point, less is more. Learn deeply and let it sit. After all, in Part 3 you will have the opportunity to bring about more sustainable changes over the course of 21 consecutive days.

THE GUT AND YOUR DIET

You're probably eager to understand how these principles can be incorporated into your diet, but I'm going to test your patience just a little more. First, let's understand the nature of the chamber that receives the diet, i.e. our gut. In my experience, the first function of food, even before nourishment or nutrients, is to protect and enhance the environment of the gut. I want you to take that very seriously. After all, food is of no use if the gut cannot welcome and use it effectively. You are not what you eat; you are only what you digest.

The Earth is believed to be home to some 8.7 million species and the gut to trillions of microorganisms that form colonies of essential microbiomes. We may be uncertain about how life first emerged on our planet or in our gut, but we know that as long as the environment and atmosphere are right, life will continue to thrive in both places and, in turn, support more life. Just as the sun, water, and atmospheric pressure keep life ticking on Earth, comparable warmth and moisture support life in our gut. Literally.

As we've seen, Ayurveda calls this warm, life-friendly environment of the gut "Agni," which directly translates as "fire." It's comparable to our systemic Inner Climate® but slightly more potent, with the ability to release transformative and warm digestive juices quickly. The dense population of microbiome that resides in the gut keeps working to support the breakdown and movement of food. About 3,000 years before the world got excited about the discovery of gut flora in the 1840s, Ayurveda stated that this very Agni is akin to life. In fact, in its prerequisites for health, Agni is listed second only to doshic balance in importance, which, again, can only be achieved through a balanced Inner Climate®.

AYURVEDA'S DEFINITION OF HEALTH

Samadoṣa samāgni ca sama dhātu malakriyah
Prasanna ātma indriya manah svastha iti abhidhīyate

When all three doshas are balanced, the Agni is balanced, and thus when the formation of tissues and waste are balanced. When the Spirit, senses, and mind are fulfilled, that is when a person is said to be in good health.

Modern science today has been amazed at the role that the environment of the gut plays in our overall health, and, thus, its role in disease, including mental health, autoimmune conditions, and even neurological disorders such as Parkinson's disease. Dysbiosis of the gut (that is, an imbalance of the microbial communities inhabiting our gastrointestinal tract) takes place when there is climate change. So, if you want to be happy with your health, keep your microbiome happy. And, if you want to keep your microbiome happy, you want to think along the lines of your Inner Climate®, warm and moist – but slightly more potent.

I must clarify right away that the Agni, our digestive fire, can easily be misunderstood, creating the potential for causing greater damage. This was the case for Sasha, who discovered Ayurveda on her trip to Rishikesh, India. The local Ayurvedic doctor she visited gave his verdict: "It is your Agni that is dysfunctional; once you set your Agni right, your constipation and bloating will disappear, and disease will never dare to be in your proximity."

At the time, the movie *Eat, Pray, Love* was a hit, and people started believing that a trip to India could be a catalyst for radical personal transformation. Sasha was not far behind, and her quest led her to Dr. Google to tell her what Agni was and how she could kindle this fire. In no time, her pantry was filled with pungent, potent, so-called Agni teas full of black pepper, cayenne, and cloves; her food was loaded with fresh ginger and spice. By the time she came to see me, her main complaint was burning in her stomach and stools; her gastroenterologist had recommended she get an endoscopy and other tests to rule out ulcers.

As soon as I heard her story, I knew that she had mistaken Agni as being just about generating heat rather than an actual environment, so she'd set her gut on fire by overdosing on spices, which led to the depletion of the soft protective mucosal lining. She had turned her insides into a hot desert, not conducive to life. And in this Sasha is not alone.

I don't want you to make the same mistake. Agni is not fire that burns like a matchstick, dry and aggressive; instead, it is the flame of an oil lamp that is moderate, supported and sustained by the *moisture* of the oil, where the moist mucosal lining tames the hot acids and bile. It is both the fire and the fuel. And yes, while certain herbs and specific foods can enhance this life-supporting environment, they are often not sustainable. It's simpler to maintain and sustain your Agni by simply following two rules based on the three principles. These are not only universal and easy to follow, but liberating.

Rule # 1: Eat Warm and Moist

The *Charaka Samhita,* the oldest known Ayurvedic text, has a detailed section on dietetics that enumerates 10 guidelines for food consumption. Though they will all make their way into this book directly or indirectly, the first two answer our question for now:

- Consume warm foods.

- Consume moist foods.

I know you're not surprised. But what does this really mean? Just how do you bring in warmth and moisture?

Bring in Warmth

If you can check the following three boxes, you've successfully brought *warmth* into your foods: cooked, freshly warm, and spiced. While I recommend including all three elements in each main meal as much as possible, skipping one or the other is fine when it comes to snack time.

Cooked

Raw foods are celebrating their heyday, but I suspect this fad would make your grandmother wince. Can you imagine yourself thriving for long in a forest full of fruits and raw meat from dead animals if you ever found yourself stranded in the wild? You may survive but not thrive; the truth is that we only evolved into this unique, robust species when we began to use fire to cook our foods. It is precisely this that makes us less wild, less primitive, more human and smarter than our apish counterparts.

Raw foods consume a lot of energy to start the breakdown process. If you left raw broccoli sitting on your kitchen counter and forgot about it for a couple of days, you'd probably return to a wilted and withered vegetable, but it wouldn't be drastically different from its original form. However, if you left cooked broccoli out on the counter for the same period, you would probably come back to a rapidly broken down, decayed, smelly mess. But this exact ability to break down quickly when cooked is a gift to the gut. Cooking activates the Agni present in the foods and the foods have little choice but to keep breaking down. And luckily for us, our gut microbiome allows for the extraction of nutrients and nourishment, eliminating the waste material as fecal matter. So we can take advantage of the rapid metabolism that cooked foods support, but without the decay.

Research supports this Ayurvedic claim. Studies have revealed that the act of cooking, encompassing not just the application of heat but physical methods such as chopping and grinding, effectively lightens the body's digestive burden.[3] This allows us to extract more energy from our food while conserving the energy usually needed for digestion. By breaking down the tough collagen in meat and softening the cell walls of plants, cooking liberates their essential nutrients, such as starch and fat.

It is this nutritional boost that is believed to have powered the development of larger brains in our early human ancestors and reduced the need for energy-hungry tissues in their guts. It is exactly what makes us human. This fascinating transition can be observed in the evolutionary shift from the broad-trunked physiques of apes to the slimmer waists characteristic of Homo sapiens, showcasing the profound impact of cooking on our evolution. I suspect that if we fed cooked food to chimps, they would, in a few million years, be building their own civilizations.

Raw salads aren't gut-friendly; however, they can be safely consumed with the added warmth of black pepper or vinegar and the moisture of a good quality oil (see page 000 for more on these). Eat them as a small side portion for lunch, preferably in the warmer months.

Freshly warm

This means consuming foods soon after they are cooked, while they are still warm, ideally from stove to table to tummy within 48 minutes. The sum of 48 minutes is the amount of time it takes according to Ayurveda for bacteria to start to grow, slowly at first and then rapidly, which is not too far off the modern-day two-hour rule. If food is kept overnight, the growth of undesirable bacteria becomes exponential. However, we have found a way to extend the life of our cooked foods by refrigerating them, putting them in a state of temporary coma by shutting down their very life processes. Ayurveda calls this a loss of *prana,* and food must possess prana if it is to support our human life force or prana in turn.

Prana answers the question, "How much life have you got in you?" Prana is that life force, the subtle energy that distinguishes the animate from the inanimate. (The concept of qi in traditional Chinese medicine is comparable to prana.) It's what leaves our body with our last breath. When we rest and regulate, we enhance prana, whereas prana becomes feeble when we are depleted. When foods are refrigerated, their prana is drastically diminished. Life is no longer ticking at the same rate in them. When foods are left overnight, the prana in them can be compromised. No wonder it's become harder for us to derive nutrients from our food.

The breath carries prana into the minutest channels of the body, and its flow can be blocked or impeded when organs are diseased, or trauma of any sort is stored in the body. When you feel alive, refreshed, and balanced and can show up for life fully, chances are that your prana is vital. However, consistent fatigue and hopelessness indicate weak prana. This life force is flowing at its best when your solar and lunar energies are aligned.

That being said, I understand that our "farm-to-table" lives have been downgraded to "work and eat at the table," and cooking is a luxury for many. And I must accept this reality if I'm to ask you to make any changes. So I'd like to suggest the generous use of Crock-Pots and slow cookers, Instant Pots and air fryers, easy stir-fry recipes, stews and even eating out at places where they serve freshly made food and the turnover is high. You can even cook in the morning and then keep food stored warm in a thermos, or with the warm setting of an electric cooker. Given our time-deprived lives, it's even OK if you need to reheat it once before consumption, as long as this is on the same day. Wait till the next day, and it becomes officially stale.

Right now, this approach may seem very ambitious, but I'm almost certain that you'll become a fan once you experience the bounty of fresh food and the joy of cooking. Not only that, when you touch, transform, and get intimate with the ingredients in your kitchen, you'll learn about them intuitively and reform your relationship with food as a result. If we can find time to exercise, we can find at least a third of that time to cook.

Rachel, a corporate lawyer living in Omaha, had never cooked in her 43 years. Her defense was that her mother was a first-generation immigrant and had never cooked, and nor had her four sisters. Her late Estonian grandmother may have cooked, but she had never witnessed it. Cooking was just not part of their family culture.

Rachel came to me in March 2022 for help with her severe inflammation, which had led to rheumatoid arthritis. She bought her meals from food stations at the grocery store in the form of frozen packaged dinners and commercial baked goods, and her preferred forms of hydration were soft drinks, black coffee, and vodka cocktails on Fridays. I was grateful that she didn't have it worse.

Home-cooked dinners were non-negotiable for me, so as part of our contract to work together, I shipped her a small electric multi-cooker, a vegetable chopper, a basic collection of spices, and a jar of ghee. She started out by making simple soups from my soup recipes e-book. Within a few weeks, she had mastered minestrone, chili, barley, and lentil soups. She then summoned up the courage to make rice-based dishes. By Thanksgiving, Rachel sent me pictures of the healthy feast she'd cooked for her sisters. Her message read, "I cannot thank you enough for the gift of cooking and the shift it's made." If cooking is foreign to you, like it was for Rachel, it can feel daunting at first, but if you take baby steps and keep at it with simple recipes, it becomes intuitive and fun.

There are exceptions to this rule, such as fruits that have been pre-ripened by the sun and certain soft vegetables like tomatoes and cucumber. We'll take a look at these later in the book. Another process that eliminates the need for cooking is fermentation. The very act of fermentation thrives on warmth and moisture; thus the macrobiotic revolution. But too much fermented food can make the gut acidic, so fermented foods are best consumed in small portions or as sides like kimchi and Ayurvedic pickles. For now, start actively thinking about where you can free up 20 to 30 minutes in the first half of your day so that you are ready to cook by the time you reach Part 3.

One more thing – don't unplug your refrigerator and use it as a closet just yet. It can still be used to store uncooked food materials like fresh fruit, vegetables, milk, jams, and condiments, for example.

Did you know that fermented foods support the probiotic environment? I want you to think about the two main properties of fermentation. It is an exothermic process, meaning that it generates heat as a by-product of chemical reactions. Most fermentation chemical reactions also release water molecules. So if you have ever fermented anything, you've probably witnessed this warmth and moisture.

Spices

This is a good time for me to tell you that warmth is not always about something's temperature. Foods can be inherently warm and if you tune in to your intuition, you can probably tell. For example, even room-temperature coconut water can feel cooling, while even a refrigerated habanero chili can feel hot. While you don't need to know the inherent properties of all foods, we'll talk about important food groups and their distinctive qualities throughout the book.

All that being said, where do you think spices rank on the scale of cool to hot? It's fair to say that spices are a crafty, effective, and delicious way of adding warmth to your foods. Ayurvedic recipes are loaded with spices for this very reason. In fact, almost every traditional Ayurvedic recipe starts with whole spices (warmth) being tempered and activated in a warm good fat, usually ghee (moist). (I will talk more about harmful fats in Part 3, page 186.)

While the world has taken to spices such as turmeric, we are still far from comprehending their full benefits, especially when used in cooking. Spices, in general, help break down foods, enhance digestive fire, and support the metabolism of fats. Each unique spice has additional benefits, such as hormonal regulation, assimilation of foods, or breakdown of plaque, to name a few examples. (See the table on page 193 for my recommended list of spices, their uses and benefits.) Unfortunately, new Ayurveda converts often confuse spices for meaning everything spicy, as Sasha did. These can be quite different. As was the case for poor Sasha, very spicy foods can often set your gut on fire, drying out the moist mucosal lining and leaving your insides feeling like they were trapped in a forest fire, rather than cozy warmth.

A good spice is one that you can find in the spice aisle of grocery stores, but doesn't feel too intense on your tongue. For this reason, cinnamon, cumin, and coriander are all examples of good spices. If a spice erodes your saliva and chars your tongue, chances are that it may do the same thing to your gut's mucosal lining. You can eat more pungent spices by making sure that they are well diluted by a good fat or food.

Bring in Moist

While cooking breaks down food and, as a result, releases moisture, it takes more than just this to meet the gut's moisture requirements. Ayurveda recommends that if the gut were divided into three parts, one-third should be filled with solid food, one-third with liquid, and one-third should be left vacant for easy movement of substances. The reference to liquid doesn't mean that we should gulp down liquids, but rather ensure that both moist and dry components make it into our foods in roughly equal parts. In fact, almost all healthy comfort foods have this consistency. For example, the famous Ayurvedic kitchari – a dish made from rice and lentils – is similarly semi-solid.

Two things are specifically important when bringing in moisture: choosing naturally moist foods and using good fats.

Choose naturally moist foods

As far as possible, choose naturally moist foods like cooked grains, avocados, sweet potatoes, zucchini (aka courgette), squashes, coconuts, and ghee, for example, versus dry and diet foods like dry crackers, cauliflower rice, and lentil pasta. Not only are the latter gut-unfriendly due to their dry nature, but they're highly processed most of the time. But if you occasionally find drier foods appealing, let these be accompanied by moist additions, like drier crackers with a creamy tahini topping, or popcorn with butter, for example.

Use of good fats

As mentioned earlier, every Ayurvedic recipe starts with good cooking fat and spices – that's our "warm and moist" right there, the very first step of food preparation. After shying away from fats for many years, modern-day nutritionists are now making a U-turn and are beginning to acknowledge as well that good fats are essential for the gut, cell building, and the nervous system.

Fats also serve as fuel for the Agni and help to keep your food breaking down at an even rate in your digestive system. You may also find it interesting to know that the Sanskrit Ayurvedic word for digestion is the same as cooking, *Paak*. Most rules that apply to cooking also apply to digestion. For example, imagine trying to roast chopped potatoes in the oven without any oil or butter on them... They would come out dry, unevenly cooked and perhaps even charred.

In the Ayurvedic world, the good fat would ideally be ghee. If you've ever hung out in the aisles of wellness grocery stores, which I suspect you have, you've probably met this hero, the latest superstar in the superfood world, but present for 5,000 years in the Ayurvedic world. So what is ghee, and why should you consider using it?

Often known as gut butter, ghee was the original omega-3 before the term "omega-3" was even coined. Sourced from whole cow's milk traditionally, it's the stuff that yogis' guts and nerves thrive on. So why is this animal-sourced fat making news in today's plant-based times? The answer lies in the fact that ghee comes from a mammal's milk, and human bodies are experts at utilizing a mammal's milk to generate new cells and create protective lining in the body. A newborn can grow significantly and survive on just its mother's milk (also a mammal). Since we constantly need raw material for new cells, what better than ghee?

Ghee contains the best of milk and leaves out the not-so-friendly aspects like casein and lactose, as these are mostly removed in the process of making ghee. Casein is the protein that makes milk heavy and hard to digest by adults, while lactose is the sugar in milk that many are intolerant to. The cherry on top is that traditional ghee is always cultured, which means that an added dose of warmth and moisture through fermentation is added to it. In fact, it is the only fat that Ayurvedic texts literally address as *Deepana* or fuel to the digestive fire.

While research on it is limited, the Ayurvedic community also strongly believes that women who consume ghee have a lower need for HRT, as well as a lower chance of developing neurological disorders. If you choose to moisten your life with ghee, make sure you buy ghee of the highest quality. It should be made from whole milk if possible; if not, from organic non-homogenized dairy. But if animal products are not for you, then don't worry – I've got you covered in Part 3.

I don't recommend that you start cooking all your foods in ghee overnight. It should be introduced slowly so that your body can become accustomed to it and learn how to utilize it effectively.

> If we spent the same amount of time we spend talking and reading about health in our kitchens actually cooking, we would soon solve most of our health concerns.

Rule # 2: Eat with the Cycle of the Sun

Have you ever eaten a heavy meal at night and found yourself tossing and turning in bed, knowing that the same meal, if consumed during the daytime, would have been much more forgiving? Well, our bodies know how to dance to the circadian rhythms; our intellectual minds are just catching up. I'm going to reiterate here that simply tuning in to and following the natural peaks and decline in our metabolic ability according to the cycle of the sun alone can be a huge game changer. Setting one body clock right can have a domino effect and set off all other body clocks in the right direction, including bowel movements, menstrual cycles, and sleep.

So what does eating with the sun look like? Well, it looks like a light, warm, and nourishing breakfast that is ideally enhanced by a spice to offset the sogginess of the morning and get you through the first few hours of the day.

The idea of "breakfast like a king" doesn't hold true and, in fact, is fairly recent, dating back only to the mid-20th century. I suspect it came about to make workdays longer and increase productivity as the world moved toward industrialization. A big breakfast significantly slows down the body, and as a result, peak metabolic activity is never achieved. Instead, breakfast should be such that it is easily digested by noon so your Agni is ready and fired up for the meal with the largest allowance, lunch. Eat lunch till you are around 70 percent full, so your food has space to keep moving through the digestive system. If a post-lunch lull is your concern, you will be surprised that as you start eating a lighter and warmer breakfast, your lunch will begin to feel more energizing instead of creating sluggishness.

As the sun begins to set, so does our Agni. We were never meant to be this dinner-eating species that we've evolved into. So dinner for an average adult is meant to be early and light, as close to 6pm as possible. I don't recommend staying up too long after the clock strikes 9.30, but if you do and if you get hungry, a hot and spiced cup of milk will do the trick.

Here are some sample menus that will help you to make sense of how these tenets can be applied (see Appendix 1 on page 255 for recipe details):

Breakfast
Principle: warm, light, mildly fatty, and preferably spiced
Main idea: anything cooked and spiced
Sourdough toast with olive oil or ghee
Steel-cut oatmeal (coarse oatmeal) or porridge with cinnamon
Hot spiced milk with almonds (soaked in water overnight and peeled)
Cooked apples with cinnamon and/or cloves
Roasted sweet potatoes with rosemary or other herbs

Lunch
Principle: largest meal, always cooked, spiced, and made with good fats
Main idea: mixed bowls work really well (indulge yourself now if you are going to anything else)
Rice and beans with a side of veggies
Asian fried rice with veggies in black bean sauce
Rice and lentils bowl with veggies or kitchari

Sushi with side of dumpling soup
Mixed bowls (Mediterranean, Lebanese, Indian, Asian,
    Mexican, etc.)
Tacos with beans and veggies
Falafel sandwich in warm pita
Sandwich in sourdough bread with a side of lentil soup
Chili with toast

Dinner
Principle: half the amount of lunch, light and cooked
Main idea: Simple, light, and super clean
Vegetable soup and stir-fry
Minestrone soup with cannellini beans
Lentil soup and a piece of sourdough
A small side of rice with veggies
Savory buckwheat pancake and a small soup
A small portion of kitchari

Well, I don't expect you to make all these changes overnight, and I will guide you through them day by day in Part 3. But for now, I want you to let the larger picture settle in: warm, cooked, and fresh foods, always paired with good fats and spices, and consumed in accordance with the sun.

At this point, you may have begun to wonder how these principles can be applied to fruit, caffeine, alcohol, raw foods, water, and the like. I want you to try to answer that yourself: Become really curious and see what you come up with. The question you really want to ask is how to feel this intuitively. Let's use the example of caffeine. Do you think caffeine is heating to the system? Do you think it's drying? Did you think of the word "dehydrating"? Literally hot and dry? Just sit with these inquiries for now. This will help you to prime your mind to think in an Ayurvedic way, making you the ultimate expert.

EXERCISE

I feel confident that most people will agree that exercise is important, regardless of whether they practice it. But I doubt most people know exactly why or how to exercise for their specific body type, or when, or even how much to exercise. The people I meet often exercise either too little, their bodies sluggish and stagnant, or too much and too hard to the point of depletion and injury, like Adrienne, the Harvard burned-out ex-lawyer I met at yoga class.

Let's return to our body's ideal warm and moist Inner Climate®, where all fluids traverse the system's channels, passing through narrow paths, and making complex turns to reach all of the body's extremities in perfect flow. Systemically, the blood, plasma, and lymph supply and transport oxygen, nutrients, hormones, proteins, white blood cells, amongst other things, and carry out excesses and unwanted substances throughout the body. What an impeccable distribution system and waste management system! However, when the body slows down and becomes sedentary, so does this system. The Inner Climate® becomes humid and dense, circulation suffers, and channels get blocked, perhaps even leading to an accumulation of sorts and depriving organ systems of their essentials. Often, people who don't exercise will experience the heaviness that accompanies this.

At the very least, exercise warms up the system, loosens all that is stagnant and stuck, and allows the body's transportation network – aka the circulation – to keep flowing, ensuring that there is no traffic jam and that all organs get their required juices. This is even more important today as humans spend more time freezing at their desks rather than moving on their farmlands. But even during our farming days, around 5,000 years ago, Ayurveda deemed that exercise was important for almost everybody.

Besides the enhanced agility, range of movement, and improved circulation that exercise brings, it causes friction and heat in the body that allow for the breakdown of excess tissue, especially unhealthy fat tissue. Fat tissue is stubborn and dense and serves as an important resource for energy when stored in the right places and in the right quantities. But when it begins to accumulate unnecessarily, it effects the warm and moist climate, making the environment too humid and dense. Thus, high cholesterol, high blood pressure, and diabetes are likely to ensue. In contrast, the heat from exercise breaks down fat cells, which are then mostly converted into energy. Moreover, exercise leads to the sculpting and strengthening of the body. Yet it nevertheless requires precaution and consideration. Get ready to hear me contradict everything you have ever heard about intense exercise ...

The Two Ayurvedic Rules of Exercise

Let's face it, exercise is a solar activity that moves the body toward the hot and dry spectrum. Just like everything solar, it needs to be done with caution, or the Inner Climate® can quickly become hot and dry, leading to depreciation and decline. That is true, especially for those who are already leaning in that direction. But if you pick your exercise wisely and support your body as recommended by Ayurveda, you'll be a winner. For those who are on the other side of the spectrum and are more lunar, dense, over-nourished, and more sluggish, exercise is thy medicine.

Rule #1: Exercise to Half of Your Capacity

Ayurveda's first rule for exercise is not to push yourself beyond your limits, but that it should be done to half of your capacity. Now, my capacity for exercise could be different from yours, so how do we quantify this subjective metric? Well, Ayurveda takes the guesswork out of it and states that when droplets of perspiration appear on your forehead and you become breathless, your body has generated enough heat, and you've reached the tipping point of solar. Anything beyond this can affect the precious soft tissues. The goal is to build up your lung capacity, heart rate variability and endurance so that your breaking point can be gradually delayed and you can exercise for longer periods.

Rule # 2: Meals Should be Oily and Contain Good Fats

When it comes to anything drying, Ayurveda's approach is almost always defensive. A dry Inner Climate® can be like an arid autumn in the human body, and quickly moves us toward barren winter, when a reversal to spring and summer (that is, youth) can be challenging. I've seen clients miss their periods and compromise their fertility due to harsh exercise regimens combined with fat-conservative diets. The fact is: Exercising more + Eating less = Being Overworked + Undernourished. How can this formula be conducive to life?

Since exercise is solar, it's fair to assume that it will heat and eventually dry the body over a period of time in those who don't carry excess body tissue. Thus, the second rule is that we must consume foods with good fats on exercise days. When we're actively burning body fat through exercise, good fats protect the essential soft tissues. Let me explain what I mean: The body doesn't just burn in parts, and when unwanted body fat is burning, so are moist tissues and substances that protect the nerves and support the joints, hold the ovum, coat the gut lining, and even provide moisture to hair follicles. An aggressive weight-loss plan loaded with exercise but conservative on good fats leads to insomnia, anxiety, bloating, hair loss, and even missed periods, as was the case for my client Leela.

Leela was based in London, and even though I saw her only behind a screen, her dry eyes, dry hair, and gaunt face told me all I needed to know about her depleted state. Her below-average BMI of 17 gave me the same story. Her periods had been irregular for the last six years, and had completely disappeared for the past three to four months. I could tell that she was a little hesitant about sharing her history, perhaps even annoyed at the prospect of introspection.

After building up trust with her, she finally revealed that she had been on one exercise and diet plan after another, each one more depleting. The most recent regime entailed her showing up at the gym at 5.30 am six days a week for 40-minute intense sessions. It'd also been recommended that she did two back-to-back 40-minute sessions on two of the five days. As prescribed, she also consumed cold soy yogurt for breakfast, uncooked sprouts, and tofu with a sprinkling of dressing for lunch, and a protein pancake for dinner. Her friends marveled at her dedication, but the truth was that she had stopped loving her body, her food, and her life.

It took a lot of counseling and the introduction of healthy new rituals for us to rebuild her relationship with food. I added good fats and some herbs to her diet, and moderated her exercise regimen. And lo and behold! Within the next quarter, her bowel movements were regular, her menses made their reappearance, and she was generally much happier and healthier. Leela had a new-found appreciation for the couple and a half pounds that now cushioned her body and protected her insides. She even remarked that her clothes actually fit better, and people noticed her radiance.

To reiterate, consuming moderate amounts of good fats may seem counterintuitive for someone who exercises with the goal of burning body fat, but it's an essential lunar replenishment for your lunar juices and could help you avoid burnout. This doesn't mean increasing your fat intake excessively, but ensuring that you are consuming regular amounts of healthy fats as part of your diet.

However, if you are already over-nourished and consume large quantities of fat regularly, you're an exception to this rule. In that case, you can significantly lower your fat intake and switch to healthier fat options for the amount you need to exercise.

When You Exercise Matters

While you want to balance the solar aspects of exercise with appropriate lunar inputs, you certainly don't want to exercise in the evening, a time when your body is transitioning into the planet's lunar phase and settling down for rest and repair. Exercising in the evening can easily stimulate the mind and body, making it harder to fall asleep.

This leaves you with the three main slots from the solar phase for exercise:

- 6am to 10am – the Juicy Morning Hours

- 10am to 2pm – the Hot Midday Hours

- 2pm to 6pm – the Windy Early Evening Hours

The midday hours between 10am and 2pm are too hot in many parts of the world to engage in an activity that builds even more heat. Exercising during these times can aggravate the nervous system and gut, even making you hangry. That crosses out midday as an option. Let's examine the afternoon hours of 2pm and 6pm, by the end of which the body and mind feel naturally depleted from the daytime solar activities and seek to unwind. Exercise during these hours may release endorphins that can perk your mood and even give you a second wind of energy, but this can be a disservice to the body, which has already expended its essential moisture. So unless your exercise takes the form of a gentle walk in nature, which is a fine balance between solar and lunar, this phase is also a no-go for exercise on a regular basis.

That leaves us with the juicy morning hours between 6am and 10am, when the body is transitioning from night to day and could use a little solar spark to propel it forward. This makes it the ideal time to exercise. Moving your body in this phase also helps bring down the rising blood sugar and cortisol levels. That being said, I acknowledge that in our individualistic, DIY lives, mornings can feel like a storm, and this can feel like a big ask. But I'm not asking you to do it all overnight. Join me in Part 3, and I will help you bring in the shifts gradually and organically.

Male and Female Bodies Experience Exercise Differently

Let's address the elephant in the room: I'd like our conversation to set aside issues of gender equality and sexuality for a moment to embrace the undeniable biological distinctions between bodies. Those assigned male at birth are naturally endowed with higher levels of testosterone, the hormone that allows them to have muscular, sculpted bodies that resonate with solar energy – traits that historically positioned them as hunters within our societies. Thus, the male pursuit for a harder body is only natural.

Those assigned female at birth, in contrast, embody the lunar essence with their softer, more yielding forms. They are graced with the nurturing gifts of soft breasts, the miraculous capacity to create amniotic fluid and breastmilk, and the tender vulnerability of easily shedding tears. To preserve the female essence, their bodies are meant to be softer and not to harden easily, even upon exercise.

Also consider this: Male sperm, unable to withstand the warmer conditions of the male body, find sanctuary in the cooler confines of the testes, ingeniously situated outside the torso. Meanwhile, the female body not only provides a safe haven for sperm but also energizes them, guiding them on their critical journey toward the egg. This highlights a universal truth: Moisture is essential for fertility, a principle that holds true across all life. And the preservation of moisture and softness is the preservation of fertility.

Pro-tip for Protein

Martha shook her head and said wistfully, "I feel like my body is no longer tender. I've lost all my feminine attributes and am starting to look like my twin brother." While Martha said this to me in a lighthearted way, her concern was obvious. At the age of 27, she had developed polycystic ovary syndrome (PCOS), a condition that came with its own entourage: androgens or male hormones, a male-pattern baldness, and hirsutism – wiry hair in unwanted places.

Her plea and frustration were both justified. She had done everything recommended by the nutritionists at her gym, almost to the T, and yet still she suffered. However, the problem lay not in her compliance but in the prescription. Copious amounts of protein powders and heavy weights had become part of her daily routine, and I felt sorry for her plight and for the plight of the millions of other women like her who succumb to fashionable but unsustainable ideas around exercise.

The case for women to protect their softness has already been made in this chapter, so this transition to protein feels like an organic next step to tackle. People consume protein for its enhanced muscle-building properties, which, in sudden large doses, can hurt female fertility. Fertility isn't just about your ability to conceive; it's also an important indicator of health during your youth. It's representative of your body's vitality and ability to sustain life.

I'm not saying that you need to give up protein. Protein is important for several body functions. However, I'm not going to be gung-ho about you becoming gung-ho when it comes to consuming proteins in isolation and increasing your protein intake suddenly. Proteins are very heavy to break down and always need to be cooked well and paired with good fats and spices.

Rather, let proteins enter your diet organically every single day. Try chili made with black beans, lentil soups, pinto bean tacos, soaked almonds as a breakfast accompaniment, tahini in your falafel, and cottage cheese with spices. Or enjoy a traditional sattu shake, like the one in the recipe below – the OG Ayurvedic protein drink designed to be easy to break-down to balance the body.

Sattu Shake

When you want an added boost, try this traditional Ayurvedic sattu drink. No surprise that it's served warm and paired with spices. The version with the buttermilk is delicious. However, I wouldn't recommend you drink this more than three times a week unless your Agni is at its best game.

Cook time: 5 minutes
Serves: 1

Ingredients

1 cup (9fl oz/250ml) water
¼ cup (1oz/30g) sattu (roasted chickpea flour)
1 tablespoon ghee or coconut oil
½ teaspoon ground cumin
½ teaspoon ground ginger (or a small piece of fresh ginger, grated)

¼ teaspoon black salt (kala namak) or regular salt
A pinch of turmeric powder (optional)
Fresh herbs like cilantro (coriander) or mint, chopped, to
    garnish (optional)

Method
1. Warm the water in a kettle until hot but not boiling.
2. In a bowl, combine the sattu with a small amount of the
    warm water to make a smooth paste.
3. In a saucepan, heat 1 tablespoon of ghee or coconut oil
    over medium heat.
4. Gradually add the sattu paste to the oil in the saucepan,
    stirring continuously to avoid lumps, then add the
    remaining warm water.
5. Return the mixture to the heat and stir constantly until it
    thickens a bit and is heated through.
6. Stir in the cumin, ginger, salt, and a pinch of turmeric
    powder, if using.
7. Mix well and gently heat for an additional minute.
8. Pour the sattu drink into a mug.
9. Garnish with fresh herbs if desired.
10. Enjoy immediately.

Tip: You can also use Ayurvedic buttermilk instead of the
        water for this sattu shake. Just make sure to stir
        constantly so it doesn't curdle.

Exercise is Solar

To sum up, exercise is a solar activity. It warms up the system,
promotes circulation, chisels the body into shape, improves
your mood, and gets your juices flowing. Exercise is also a
great way to burn excess body fat, with the caveat that it
may burn up essential soft tissues for those with moderate
to lean bodies. So your recommended daily dose will depend

on your excesses. Those who've stayed away from exercise the longest usually need it the most, but get there gradually. Bringing intention and restraint into how hard you push your body and supporting your body with good fats is Ayurveda's antidote for the potential ill effects of exercise.

SLEEP

Food, medicine, exercise, and therapy – all of them combined cannot do what a good night's sleep can for the body and mind. Sleep is our ultimate opportunity for daily rest, recovery, and healing: nighttime slumber temporarily halts depreciation and is one of Ayurveda's three pillars or prerequisites for health (good nutrition and appropriate use of bodily fluids through sexual self-restraint being the other two). You may also remember from Part 1 that the glymphatic system, which flushes out debris accumulated from nervous activity, is most active at nighttime when the body is asleep. Not only that, substances like growth hormone and prolactin surge to help build new cells and regulate immunity. Your own body has a healing center that welcomes you to take advantage of it every single night!

How can this be understood through the lens of the Inner Climate®? Well, everything that keeps your body burning during the day – like work, exercise, stress, caffeine, productivity, conversation, and movement – shuts down during the hours of sleep so the body can be refueled at night. My choice of words is deliberate here: "burning in the day" and "refueled" at night. "Burning" denotes the dry and hot effect of the solar phase as well as solar activities, while "refueled" is indicative of the moistening that happens as a result of nighttime sleep. Burnout, inflammation, heat rashes, exhaustion, burning in the eyes, skin sensitivity, and acidity are not uncommon for those who cannot balance their daytime burn with nighttime sleep and other lunar activities. Similarly, if you stay in bed longer than required and nap at odd hours, your body is going to retain extra moisture, clog your insides, and make you sluggish and sedentary. But, when the burning and refueling happen at a proportionate rate, the body can restore its ideal warm and moist Inner Climate®.

The Right Time to Sleep

The right time to sleep is not when your dinner has shifted you into a state of coma, or when you're too tired to stay up, or when you've finally completed those deadlines. The right time to sleep is determined by your master clock, the suprachiasmatic nucleus (SCN) located in your hypothalamus. The SCN relies upon two clocks to regulate our sleep and wake cycles.

The exogenous clock, or nature's clock, relies on environmental cues like darkness and light to create sleep–wake patterns. The eyes sense darkness and the body prepares to sleep, and vice versa. For thousands of years of thriving human evolution, in the eras before electricity and before the age of travel through time zones, our SCN heavily relied on this clock. Not only did it allow us to regulate our sleep cycles according to the time of day and the seasons, but it allowed us to align our digestion and hormonal rhythms according to universal design, thus enjoying natural balance and flow.

The endogenous clock is an internal biological clock that relies on our personal behaviors and patterns to induce sleep and wake cycles, independent of whether our eyes experience darkness or light. This is an important clock, especially during short winter days and long summer days where relying on darkness and light may not always afford us sufficient stimulation or rest. For example, if you were in Iceland at the summer solstice, experiencing sunlight for a

24-hour period, and your body relied only on the exogenous clock, you would find yourself "owl-ing" all night. But since the endogenous clock remembers the body's personal sleep cycle, it can still pump sleep-time juices into your system so you can reclaim your rest at night. By that same token, if you travel to a completely different time zone, you can blame the endogenous clock for your jet lag.

If we allowed our SCN to rely on nature's exogenous clock during days and nights of regular length and the endogenous clock for seasonal variations in the length of the day, our sleep cycles would be good as gold. We would be living in harmony with nature's design, thus thriving according to nature's plans. But in our quest for exploration and growth, we've transcended the natural boundaries of circadian rhythms and time zones. We've elongated our daytime through artificial lighting and shortened our nights in the name of productivity. Our endogenous clock has become used to erratic schedules.

For example, if you were to stay up celebrating your birthday at midnight, the adrenaline from the excitement may trump the cues from the darkness outside and allow you to remain awake longer than your body was designed to do. Or if you're working night shifts, your SCN would take cues from your endogenous clock and start delaying your sleep cycle, making it increasingly easy for you to stay up later. However, over a period of time, such shifts in patterns can be detrimental and have a domino effect on all the other cycles in the body, including digestion and menstrual cycles. In saying this, I don't mean to burden you with an unhealthy dose of complaints and warnings, but rather present my plea for us to reset our clocks to ease the load on our bodies.

Now, let me cut to the chase and get to the actual timings. Assuming that sunrise and sunset take place at approximately 6.30am and 6.30pm, we can aim to be in bed three hours or one *prahar* (which is a Sanskrit unit of time amounting to three hours) after sunset, which means 9.30pm, and perhaps be asleep by 10pm. The demands of modern-day life may not always be conducive to this schedule, but you nevertheless should try to adhere to a time that is as close to this as possible, most days a week.

Winding down during the *prahar* between sunset and bedtime is essential if you want to be able to enjoy deep and effective slumber. I recommend an evening ritual, dimming the lights, playing classical music, and even engaging in some form of introspection. Journaling right before bedtime can help you not only sleep deeper but will allow your brain to process and assimilate the events and emotions from the day.

If you've successfully managed an earlier bedtime, waking seven to eight hours later is ideal and enough sleep for most. Sleeping longer than required means overdoing the growth phase and inviting sluggishness. By the same token, sleep deprivation means losing the opportunity to repair the wear and tear of the solar phase and will invite dryness. Less growth means more transformation and decline throughout the day. In both these scenarios, we inevitably drift away from the warm and moist climate our body seeks.

What about the Night Owls?

"There's no such thing as a night owl unless you really are an owl or a bat or a tiger or another member of the nocturnal world," I said, but I could tell that Linda didn't find my statement funny. In fact, I'm not sure I intended it to be.

Linda was above average at sticking to her routines, but it was the timing of her routines that triggered her irregular periods, volatile weight, and mild depression. She rose out of bed each day at 8.30am, emptied her bowels after a cup of black coffee, went directly to the gym and then made it to her work by 11am. She left work around 8pm after the last round of students had left the testing center where she worked.

Dinner and Netflix were integral parts of her nightly routine before she retired to bed around 1am.

One could argue that Linda slept for a good number of hours and even exercised, and her symptoms seemed bizarre. However, I was eventually able to convince her to move her day just a couple of hours ahead, even if it meant watching part of her shows in the morning. She instantly felt more energetic in the mornings and had no desire to watch TV. She was occasionally even able to empty her bowels without the coffee. Her real shift came when she applied for an earlier shift at work, starting her day at 9 and ending by 6. Dinner was moved to 6.30pm, and her Netflix hours were shortened to allow time for journaling. Her depression lifted almost instantly, and soon enough, her periods became more predictable and less painful. Restoring one clock helped to restore all her clocks.

Keeping awake for several hours after sunset means that nature's clock is in a headlock with your endogenous clock. And when nature loses repeatedly, we lose. The body consumes excess energy because it's struggling to juggle its need for internal nightly repair with trying to keep awake at the same time. This need for energy is usually met by late-night hunger pangs, which the gut is not preconditioned to digest. So, for every reason, an earlier bedtime is your friend.

Long Summer Days and Short Winter Days

Does this mean that you should go to sleep early on short winter days and then really late on long summer days? It does not. The endogenous clock comes to our rescue when the length of the day changes according to the season. Even if the sunset is much later in the day, your internal clock holds the memory of your bedtime and will support the release of sleepy juices as close to that time as possible. An exception to this are those really hot summer days, when your body may need an afternoon siesta to protect its juices. In that case, and if you're in the lucky position where you can enjoy an afternoon snooze, your bedtime can be pushed back to a later hour.

Similarly, your internal clock also ensures that you won't fall asleep at 5pm on a short winter's day. And yet, cold weather increases the body's hibernation needs; thus, moving your bedtime to a slightly earlier time can only help you in the early winter months.

Making the Morning Good

Ideally, you want to get up as close to the hour of sunrise as possible, but around 6.00am to 6.30am is a realistic target for most people to be out of bed, assuming that their bedtime is between 9.30pm and 10.00pm. Simply put, if you don't meditate, you'll want to sleep for about seven to eight hours or so, but not too much more. Meditation lowers the body's need for sleep as it takes you into deeper repair mode in a shorter period of time, so meditators can afford to have slightly less sleep than others.

How can you tell if you're sleeping longer than required? If your sleep patterns are making you feel sluggish in the morning rather than energized, then you don't need a growth cycle that long, and I would suggest you experiment with getting up earlier. By the same token, if you wake up with a body that is tired and eyes that are dry but a mind that feels overstimulated and ready to go, you probably need more growth and repair and would benefit from sleeping longer and going to bed even earlier. I understand this may be your biggest challenge. However, a bedtime ritual and overall organization of your daily routine will slowly but steadily bring you into alignment.

For those one-off late nights, Ayurveda recommends that you sleep in a little longer, half of the sleep time that was compromised. So let's say you missed out on two hours of sleep at night; you catch up by sleeping in an hour later the next morning. But if you were to sleep in till mid-morning, your body's rhythms would inevitably be disrupted and affect your appetite, digestion, moods, and more.

For the spiritual seekers and the meditators, getting up 48 to 96 minutes before sunrise is ideal for accessing the subconscious mind and enjoying brain wave frequency patterns that exist when the mind is between awake and asleep. This is traditionally when the yogis woke in order to unravel the mysteries of their own minds and the world around them.

Do the Same Rules Apply to Napping?

You already know that an unbearably hot summer's day or living in a hot climate gives you a nap pass; hence the tradition of the siesta. Heat can trigger rapid exhaustion, loss of appetite, and even queasiness, which make both a protective nap and even a later bedtime permissible in summer. But with a few notable exceptions, napping after lunch isn't Ayurveda's idea of healthy sleep. In fact, quite the contrary. Eating is an essential growth activity, and the body needs to progress to the transforming phase right after eating to metabolize and utilize the food it has consumed. But if you send your body to sleep, yet another growth activity, digestion, halts and the food becomes undigested waste, which eventually begins to ferment in the system.

The exceptions to this rule include young children, the elderly, the weak, the frail, and the sickly, who are allowed to nap. You get it: Anyone who needs growth or who needs protection from decline has the privilege of a nap.

I could write an entire book on sleep, and I know that I've probably packed more information in here than your mind can process, but sleep on it – literally. Start noticing shifts in your inner and outer environment as the sun sets, and mindfully switch gears to "do less" and "be more" in the hours before bedtime. Experiment with an earlier bedtime and tune in to the quality of your sleep and dreams each night. Let the changes be driven by the shifts you witness and your own keen awareness, until we'll catch up again on the subject of sleep in Part 3, where I'll support you in making some systematic changes.

YOUR MINDSET AND RELATIONSHIPS

Our ancestors knew that the mind and body were deeply connected and that we are more than our physical body and five senses. We are a whole system of thoughts, feelings, breath, spirit, and consciousness, which essentially form the software for our hardware, the physical body. The software runs the programs on the hardware, and it's important for the hardware to be robust in order to respond to the software's programs. Let's break this down together.

Our experiences and interactions set off thoughts and feelings, which are expressed as sensations in the body. The sensations are evidence that the brain is triggered to bring about chemical changes in the body, which, over a period of time, affect our chemistry and the Inner Climate®. You and I both know the impact of climate change. As tempted as I am to throw in some science here and talk about the neurotransmitter shifts with different states of the nervous system, I am going to start by getting you to inquire deep within.

Take a moment and think about how anger feels in your body. If you could feel it as a climate, would it be hot? And how does stress feel? Hot and dry? Anxiety – dry? Panic? If you were stuck in a car accident, in a moment of panic, you would feel your mouth dry up, your follicles shrink, your hair stand on end, and your body tighten, far removed from a warm and moist state. In contrast, how does gratitude feel? Emotions instantly cause a corresponding physiological change in the body. And you don't need to be wired up to measure it. You can experience it just by tuning in.

Janet joined my 21-day healing program to work on her lifelong eczema and the autoimmune conditions that had crept up on her in the past year after a very stressful experience at work. Angry, intense, and passionate would describe her aptly. Perfectionism had become her coping mechanism after she lost her mother at the age of nine and was left in the care of her alcoholic father and his idealistic extended family. The committed being she was, I knew that she would dive into our inner work together with all she had.

The fact was that her life experiences and her mindset had burned her out. But she was blown away when she realized that each one of her symptoms – eczema, rosacea, the burning in her stomach, and her eye condition – had "hot and dry" written all over it. Not only that, she even described her relationship with her husband as snappy, with her mood being constantly on the edge – hot and dry.

After we'd discussed this, Janet emailed me to say, "My life has never made more sense to me. It's parched, it's burned. All of it, inside and out. I've constantly sought answers but found none till now. The sad part is that I've been trying to solve it by working harder, doing more, and becoming more solar and angry. I know now that all I need to do is go more lunar to find that state of being, or surrender. I know it will be a journey, but I feel like I can exhale now. I have my answers. I need to find a safe home in my body and let it all go. I've done too much, been too much, sought too much – phew!"

Her message was a sign that Janet had unlocked what was required. Sure enough, over the next 21 days, Janet experienced a tremendous breakthrough that extended beyond the remission of her eczema to the improvement of her relationships, her sleep, and her life as a whole.

Our Emotions and the Inner Climate®

Over the years, I've studied our emotions and the subsequent shifts they can create in the body's climate. Every single time, I have seen the shifts reflected in the body's physical landscape.

I hope you will be able to relate to the subjective study that follows, allow it to awaken your innate intelligence, and use it as a guide to forming your own mind–body connections.

Anger

I want you to think of the Hulk, a character in the Avengers comic book series and movies. Every time Bruce Banner, the brilliant scientist with a perfect disposition, becomes enraged, his body changes and bulks up, his eyes focus, and his gaze intensifies as his eyebrows furrow, his face becomes fierce, and his voice deepens – and he transforms into the Hulk. What do you think is happening to the world inside him?

Think of an angry scene from your own life: You can probably sense that your body temperature rises, your insides feel tighter, and perhaps your face becomes red, almost like your body is charged, heated, and ready to take action. These changes are triggered by a host of chemical reactions that heat up the system and deplete the lunar restful juices, evident in words like "heated, charged, flared, fierce," which are often used to describe the experience of anger.

If this were to happen every day, it would bring about a form of global warming in the body. Over time, the hot and dry climate can contribute to a host of imbalances in the physical body. The ones I have seen most often are inflammation, skin conditions, explosive bowels conditions, sleep trouble, and even cardiovascular trouble.

Stress

Before you think of the word "stress" as defining an emotional experience, I want you to think about it as a verb, often used to emphasize something; for example, "she stressed the importance of good hygiene." The word comes with a sense of emphatic passion. Physiological and psychological stress isn't too far from this. Passion and intensity – both are solar. Moderate stress can be useful and is a stimulus for action, productivity, and growth. However, over a period of time, chronic stress can leave us dry and burned out.

I remember a particularly busy period in my life. I launched a new program at work, moved homes, hosted 11 live-in guests, and planned for an imminent international trip – all in the same week. By the end of it, my body felt sore, my eyes were burning, my throat felt dry, and it hurt to use my voice. I became a 440V human being, and you wouldn't have wanted to be near me. As much as I needed to sleep, my nervous system felt short-circuited and aggravated. It was only after several yoga nidra sessions, a couple of massages, a digital lockdown, ear oiling, water sounds immersion, and alternate nostril breath work that I was able to restore my inner peace and Inner Climate®.

Anxiety

When you have a worry that cannot be delegated or dealt with, it hangs out in your nervous system instead, where it can turn into anxiety. Let me explain. When a concern presents itself, we usually do one of two things: Put it in the "action" bucket so we can do something about it, or the "surrender" bucket if it is beyond our control. For example, if I'm concerned about what my daughter is going to eat at school, I can make her a packed lunch: action. But if I'm concerned about the possible collision of our planet with a giant meteor in the year 3050, I would rather surrender that worry for now. (As an aside, a healthy response to anything is to balance action with surrender. For example, if you're concerned about a presentation at work, preparing for it with integrity and making a reasonable effort are action enough. Then, when you can surrender the outcome, you've won. You've balanced the solar in the action with the lunar of the surrender.) However, when we cannot assign the thought to either action or surrender, we usually begin to ruminate, and the thought picks up speed in the nervous system and continues to feed itself until we may reach a state of paralysis.

If you have ever felt anxiety, you have probably felt this initial rush, this speed in your chest. The experience is akin to a wind, drying and depleting the insides. It's not uncommon for chronic anxiety to manifest in symptoms of dryness, hair loss, dry eyes, bloating, and insomnia before aggravating the onset of a more serious condition.

Depression

Compared to the solar experiences of stress and anger, depression can feel like quite the opposite and keep us from acting. Depression instills heaviness in the body, disinterest in the mind and disengagement with life. It often results in sedentary life choices, like avoidance of social interaction, weight gain, substance reliance, and consumption of high-calorie foods. It thus results in a sluggish and dense Inner Climate®.

Other Emotions

I find it very useful to tune in to my body's sensations to understand how feelings can affect its current chemical reality in the short term and alter its biological reality in the long term. I'd urge you to do the same. You will notice that jealousy can feel slightly hot; fear dry; and guilt and shame heavy and sluggish. Our bodies are such incredible laboratories for any amount of research we might need to do to understand ourselves. It has all the answers we seek. We don't need to open it up and dissect it in order to learn from it. We just need to trust it.

Regulating Our Feelings

Let me clarify: I'm not trying to insinuate that feelings are bad. They are, in fact, very important in making our experience on Earth more real, rich, and fulfilling. It's the dysregulated and denied emotions that create chronic disruption in the climate inside us. Our first task is to accept any emotion that comes up, so our body can begin to feel safe with it, therefore making regulation possible as the next step.

When anger is regulated, it becomes passion. When anxiety takes your mind in a million directions, you can surrender and use that same force to unlock your creativity and courage. And jealousy can be turned into motivation; fear can be eased with faith, and depression with stimulation and hope. It's possible for us to keep coming back to a warm and moist state. Unfortunately, we are designed to stick with what's familiar, and we get addicted to our emotional realities and our imbalanced Inner Climate® till they become chronic symptoms in our physical bodies. And then we have a classic chicken and egg situation. Did it happen in the mind first or the body first?

While it's easy for me to ask you to regulate your feelings, it's unfair to do so without giving you the proper tools. So, I am going to introduce you to three emotions that will keep you swimming in the warm and moist. Practicing them every single day helps you to amplify and replicate the Inner Climate® they bring every time you find yourself feeling off-center.

Gratitude

Gratitude is a warm and moist emotion that fills the heart, instantly infusing it with abundance and flow. Can you relate to how that feels? Gratitude cannot be triggered through a mechanical or an intellectual process. And I'll be honest: Gratitude journaling did nothing for me besides making me feel more inept at feeling grateful, but I know that it may work for some. Here instead are the two things that did work for me:

- **Zooming out:** I normally recall the three core principles and marvel at the order of the universe: this cosmic arrangement that keeps our planet ticking. I'm reminded of the speck I am in this magnanimous reality, yet I am perfectly capable of having a heightened experience in this lifetime. So much is already in place for me to help me to live, think, and thrive! Wow!

- **Recalling my luck:** I always keep a list of things in my back pocket that I can draw upon to remind me of how lucky I am; it mentions my grandfather, the spiritual presence and guidance of my father, the practical wisdom of my mother, the ability to witness the journey of my two beautiful daughters, my Ayurvedic education, and small moments of overwhelming synchronicities. While your list of the things that remind you of your good fortune will look different, I'm certain there have been moments in your life when you have felt truly blessed and lucky. Write those down, feel them, memorize the feeling, and keep your list handy.

Compassion

I think we can both agree that compassion feels warm and moist, like a cozy hug. Tuning in to your own feelings and accepting them will make you more compassionate toward yourself. In this way, you can learn to brace yourself for those difficult moments and even to connect the dots to understand your triggers and their origins in the past. You may then realize that your reactions are the result of your unprocessed experiences, as you lacked the tools to deal with them. The result of showing compassion toward yourself is that you end up feeling greater compassion for everyone, a state that keeps your Inner Climate® optimum.

Love

Love and genuine affection are undeniably the warmest and most moist emotions. This is what makes love the most craved human emotion, and most of us spend our entire lives trying to be loved by others. But loving ourselves or even someone else unconditionally brings about similar chemical realities. We don't have to be on the receiving end of someone else's love to enjoy the benefits of love. Inner child or shadow work will allow you to love all parts of yourself, including the parts of yourself that you find difficult to accept.

Tools for Regulating Your Inner Climate®

Apart from practicing the three emotions, there are various tools that you can access to restore and regulate your emotional climate. Of these, regular sleep, meditation, alternate nostril breathing (a Vedic balancing breathing exercise), resonance breathing (breathing with longer exhalations), classical music, massages, routines, water sounds, aromatherapy, cognitive behavioral therapy, hugging, laughing, and dance are just a few of the tools that come to mind. You will get the opportunity to design your own toolkit later in the book.

Once you practice and familiarize yourself with what it is like to have a warm and moist emotional Inner Climate®, you will be able to call upon it at any time. I find myself summoning up the state before awkward social events and even before uncomfortable meetings; it feels like a warm sheath covering all of my being to keep it safe. I instantly become more present, secure, curious, and compassionate in all my relationships.

Relationships and the Inner Climate®

I have one last piece of evidence before I rest my case for the optimum Inner Climate®, when it comes to mindset and emotions. How do you prefer your people to be? Hot-tempered? Or cold? Hot-tempered individuals burn through their social circles in no time. And when a person is cold, there's stagnation in the relationship, and it lacks the passion and the fire needed to transform it and take it to the next stage. Warmth in relationships is what we seek to feel safe and to keep engaged and connected.

Awareness of your Inner Climate® and how it changes with social interactions and relationships will help you to identify which interactions serve you and enhance your well-being. This awareness will also highlight areas where you need to work on yourself.

The work on understanding your Inner Climate® begins with noticing the subtle shifts within you when you feel triggered in a relationship. Many of my clients describe how, even before fully realizing it, their Inner Climate® starts to change – often rushing toward a hot, dry state. For those who rely on reactivity as a coping mechanism, this can lead to sharp, impulsive responses, while those who tend to deny or numb their emotions might seek solace in sugar, food, inertia, or other substances.

If feeling this triggered is generally unusual for you, it's crucial to examine whether it's the relationship itself that is unhealthy, and to look for red flags or toxic behaviors within it. However, if you find yourself losing equilibrium consistently in all your relationships, it may point to a deeper trigger pattern within you – something that requires your attention and healing work.

Take Zila, a 28-year-old client of mine who'd recently moved to New York City from South Africa. Initially thrilled by her new life in the Big Apple, Zila's excitement waned as familiar patterns began to emerge. She quickly made friends but soon found herself feeling scrutinized, leading her to become defensive and irritable. Despite her efforts to salvage these relationships, they often deteriorated, prompting her to seek out new friends, only to repeat the cycle. Zila's experiences with her judgmental mother, with whom she had a strained relationship, had influenced her move to the US – an attempt to escape the constant feedback from her family. Through inner work, Zila came to realize that her own hypersensitivity to comments and feedback due to her childhood experiences was a significant part of the problem. Today, she is focused on healing, cultivating her own grounding warmth and moisture, rather than falling back into the blame game.

Aparna's story offers a different perspective. Aparna has been a close friend of mine for 25 years and she is one of the happiest and most positive people I know. She maintains healthy relationships and has mastered the art of setting boundaries to protect them. So, it was surprising to see her distraught when her recently divorced sister-in-law moved in with her and her husband. Aparna felt increasingly controlled, burdened by unnecessary demands, and perhaps even gas-lighted. Given her usual ability to maintain healthy boundaries, she quickly recognized the toxic patterns in this new relationship. She understood that her "hot and dry" reaction wasn't a resurfacing of past triggers but a genuine response to a current unhealthy dynamic.

The key is to observe what disrupts your inner warmth and moisture. Does it happen in every relationship or only in specific ones? Is it driven by past triggers and conditioning, or is there a legitimate red flag or threat present?

In my own journey, I've found tremendous value in identifying the patterns I need to break and the situations that are genuinely unhealthy. This awareness has also helped me recognize and navigate relationships that were toxic, allowing me to either shed them or find ways to maintain my Inner Climate® in a healthy, thriving state. Eventually, I hope to reach a point where the Inner warmth becomes a consistent state, unshakeable, irrespective of the external situation, but for now, I am working my way to it one day at a time.

DAILY RITUALS

There's no denying that routines and daily rituals bring a sense of grounding and cadence to our lives. They take us away from the grind and toil of everyday life, and offer us precious moments with our inner self that allow us to show up more for ourselves and thus our life as a whole. Without our daily rituals, many of us would start prioritizing everything outside of us, and wouldn't respect our own boundaries. This, in turn, would undermine our sense of self-worth and leave us exhausted and resentful. Daily rituals are like the daily "growth" we need so we can keep transforming rather than go into a state of decline.

The importance of daily rituals was brought home to me when I worked with a beautiful 40-year-old woman called Sana. The scent of her perfume entered my office before she did. Her hair was neatly tucked back, her lipstick perfect, and her silk blouse was creaseless. But only 40 minutes into our session, I realized that her external facade concealed a very different internal reality. Five pregnancies, three C-sections, a houseful of children under the age of 12, a busy and emotionally unavailable husband, deep resentment, high blood pressure, high cholesterol levels, and a misbehaving uterus were the reality of this immaculately turned-out woman.

Sana explained how she had barely exercised in the last 13 years; showers were a luxury squeezed into the rare spare moments of her day, and lunch was a hurried coffee and croissant on the go. Dressing up on the rare occasions that she did encounter the outside world kept the illusion of her perfect life alive. She often sat on the toilet seat and cried, yet it never once occurred to her that this was not normal – till her sister-in-law expressed alarm at the state of her dwindling body and spirit. She had taken a round of supplements prescribed by her functional medicine doctor. Sadly, her body rejected them all. She now wanted some easy, quick herbs, but I refused to work on her physical ailments with herbs till she could slow down and prioritize herself.

It took Sana several months, but she was eventually able to recruit family members to help with the children, build some supportive routines into her life, and regain some sense of equilibrium in her mind. As she started sleeping better and brought back some moisture into her Inner Climate®, her periods became regular and her overall health began to recover. She began to grow again, and her life was about to transform. When I bumped into her at a restaurant a couple of years later, her inner radiance matched her shiny external appearance. She introduced me to her husband and said, laughing, "Meet my Ayurvedic doctor and life coach, Nidhi – the woman who made my mornings and our lives better. Also, blame her for all those bottles of oil!" She went on to tell me that she was studying art to become an art dealer.

The Role of Ayurvedic Ritual

Ayurvedic rituals are more than just practices. They are designed to help you take advantage of the day's rhythm and guide you toward a more desirable Inner Climate®. In fact, ancient Ayurvedic literature is loaded with countless morning rituals that would eat into your afternoon if you were to practice them all. So here I'm going to introduce you to six of my favorite practices, which you can gradually incorporate into your day in Part 3.

Ayurvedic rituals are all about oiling, which is why I wanted to introduce you to this ancient secret: oil. The Sanskrit term for oil is *sneha*, which also means love, is telling of oil's warm and loving properties for the body. When Ayurveda talks about oil, this usually means sesame seed oil, with certain exceptions. Seeds carry a significant amount of latent heat in order to progress quickly into their growth phase, thus making them inherently warm. And the oil coming from the seeds is warm and moist. Ayurveda's idea of oiling every external surface and each orifice you can get into to create an environment where microbiome life can thrive is nothing short of genius. But there's more to oil than just that. Let's explore each of the following rituals and how they can help us to keep returning to the ideal Inner Climate®.

DIFFERENCE BETWEEN ROUTINES AND RITUALS

As you read about the daily Ayurvedic practices, I want you to start thinking about them as rituals, rather than routines. Routines seem like chores, something on a to-do, must-do list, a task you must check off to move on with your day. Rituals, on the other hand, are a full-on experience; they feel sacred and intimate and invite you to be present. One way to ritualize anything is to bring all your senses to the experience. Set up your space for the practice; use plants, nontoxic candles, aromas, crystals, and music. Before you begin, ground yourself by taking a few deep breaths to become fully present within yourself and the practice.

Tongue Scraping

This is one of the few Ayurvedic rituals that doesn't utilize oil. It takes less than 30 seconds and can stimulate Agni, enhance taste, and help you clear morning gunk from your tongue so you can enjoy a fresh day of digestion and consumption. It is exactly what it sounds like: scraping your tongue. You need a simple U-shaped metal device called a tongue scraper to perform this practice, ideally done after brushing.

Just as cooking in the kitchen can leave grease on the ceiling, digestion can leave residue in the digestive tract that accumulates as a thin film on the tongue. Additionally, an idle, closed mouth through the night gathers slime and bacteria that show up as a white coating on your tongue upon waking. If not scraped out, we end up consuming this film with our breakfast – neither tasty nor healthy. The practice of tongue scraping in the morning gets rid of this unwanted coat in an effective and simple manner.

Nasya

The nose is often overlooked in its potential to create inner balance. The only time our nostrils usually get attention is when they are blocked. But the nose is the gateway to the brain, bypassing the blood–brain barrier. This means that anything that enters the nose has direct access to the brain, and scientists are now studying the nose as a route for effective drug delivery to the brain. Just like many other current scientific discoveries, Ayurvedic science articulated this 5,000 years ago in a very specific statement: *Nasa hi Siraso dwaram,* meaning "The nose is the only gateway to the brain."

So, the time-tested and safe practice of nasya, or applying drops of herbal nasal oil to the nostrils every single day, nourishes your brain. Ayurveda believes that nasya's benefits extend beyond brain health, memory, and prevention of Alzheimer's disease, to promoting healthy sinuses and hair, reduction in headaches and allergies, and rebuilding of the microbiome in the ENT passages. You only need a bottle of Anu Taila nasya and 20 seconds of your day. Anu Taila is a unique herbal oil with specific herbs that target the health of this area of the body. However, if Anu Taila is unavailable where you live, start with plain sesame oil or look for another nasya oil. I will give you more guidance on this in Part 3. For now, get mentally comfortable with the idea of putting drops of oil up your nose; it's more comforting than you can imagine.

Abhyanga

You may have heard of abhyanga oil massage in some form or another. Ayurvedic hair and beauty brands have popularized hair abhyanga or hair oil massage. One of the essential practices of *dinacharya*, the Ayurvedic daily rituals, abhyanga entails massaging your body with oil, ideally before you jump into the shower. The first benefit of abhyanga is touch: How often do we get touched, or even touch ourselves, amidst the busyness of the modern world? Touch promotes the release of oxytocin, the cuddle hormone that instantly throws the body into the parasympathetic or "rest and digest" mode. More than anything, abhyanga helps you to restore the health of the microbiome that lives on your skin. Like nasya, you will learn more about this and other benefits of abhyanga later in the book.

Oil Swishing

Oil swishing is therapy for your oral health. Simply swishing coconut oil or sesame oil in your mouth for 5 to 10 minutes each day after tongue scraping can save you thousands of dollars at the dentist. While the scientific jury has still not given its verdict, I highly recommend you experience this. The oil again helps replenish the mouth's environment, ensuring that pathogens, bacteria, and bad breath don't stand a chance. It can also help to whiten teeth and strengthen jaw muscles.

Addy's story underscores the importance of good oral health. She developed an autoimmune condition, one that had made it impossible for her to eat most foods and caused inflammation in her joints. As she had grown up eating fresh foods according to Ayurvedic principles her entire life, it seemed unreasonable to her that she now had to deal with her new health status. She went from one doctor to another, but no one had an answer for her. She was prescribed steroids and immunosuppressants. A friend referred her to a kinesiologist for her aches and pains, and she agreed to go but without any expectation of help. She was shocked, as the skillful kinesiologist asked her about her gum health and whether she had had any treatment in recent years. It turned out that a root canal that went bad had remained unidentified, infecting her blood, and causing severe inflammation in her body: the root cause of her condition. Addy did what was required to fix the broken root canal and fully recovered from her condition. Addy's story proves that gum health affects your overall body and caring for them is more important than we think.

Nighttime Foot Massage

Traditional Chinese Medicine and Ayurveda both value the soles of the feet for their ability to manipulate and enhance prana, our life force. The feet contain *marma* points, energy centers where prana is concentrated. By massaging these points, prana can be stimulated and even released when blocked. Foot reflexology in TCM is based on a similar philosophy. Meridians that carry qi and flow through the body and its organs can be accessed through the feet.

After the solar productive phase, it is natural for prana to weaken at night. A nightly foot massage sets trapped prana free and regulates it so you can sleep and repair effectively. If you've ever experienced a foot massage, you probably know that it is a beneficial practice that relaxes your body and has the ability to promote deep sleep and reduce anxiety as well as nighttime cramps, but you are probably unaware of the more significant impact it can have on your wellness.

Alternate Nostril Breathing

This daily ritual comes from the philosophy of yoga, but I have taken the liberty to include it here since yoga and Ayurveda are close relatives. Our breath has the ability to regulate and enhance our prana. Just as the two hemispheres of the brain function differently, so our left and right nostrils carry unique pranic energies. The right nostril is believed to carry more solar, warmer energies, and the left nostril carries moister, lunar energies. I am not surprised that the liver, our highly metabolic organ, is located on the right side, and our heart and spleen are on the left. Depending on the time of day and condition of the body and mind, one or the other of the two nostrils may be more active.

The practice of alternate nostril breathing regulates prana by balancing solar and lunar and bringing you back to homeostasis – warm and moist. If you were to practice alternate nostril breathing, you would notice that it instantly brings calm and grounds you in the present moment. Moreover, regular practice can help with anxiety, ailments, hormonal imbalance, sleep, and moods. (For practical advice on how to do alternate nostril breathing, see Day 17 in Part 3, page 209.)

Until my early teens, I was a feisty, hot, and dry individual. You'd think that electricity flowed through my body at a high, irregular speed. Shortly after my 15th birthday, my father suggested that I go for a 10-day silent Vipassana retreat, and that changed my life.

During the first three days of Vipassana, I was asked to notice my breath in a non-judgmental manner during the 13-hour meditation days. As hard as this was, I noticed something peculiar. My right solar nostril was significantly more active, especially in the hot afternoons, and more so when I felt aggravated or impatient.

As the days progressed, breath awareness became a part of me, and I carried it even beyond the meditations. When I slept well, the left lunar nostril got a chance to shine, and if I were awoken by a nightmare, I would be back to the solar right. Over time, I have learned to use my breath as a clue to what is happening in my mind and body. At the same time, alternate nostril breathing has allowed me to take advantage of both – the right and the left, the warm and the moist.

These six rituals are enough and fairly easy to incorporate into our modern-day lives. I want you to think of these rituals as more than just prescriptions by an Ayurvedic doctor. As you begin to introduce them into your daily routine in Part 3, I want you to think about how they apply to the three core principles, how they make you feel, and how they affect your Inner Climate®. I want these rituals to support not just your body but to awaken your body's intelligence.

PART 3
YOUR 21-DAY HEALING PROGRAM

Welcome to the beginnings of a new you! You are ready to begin practicing. In this part of the book, I will introduce one new change to you each day and invite you to stack another one on it the next day. All in all, we will be applying the three core principles to making 21 shifts over a period of 21 days. This gradual easing-in will support you in slowly incorporating the ideas in this book, internalizing each shift, and keeping your efforts sustainable. So, at the end of 21 days, you would have made 21 shifts. This may sound ambitious, but it's mostly about reconfiguring and rearranging your life according to the principles and making choices different from the ones you've probably been making so far. Most of the shifts won't demand any extra time from you or eat into your day. Also, once you internalize the three principles, the choices feel organic.

Twenty-one also happens to be the number of days it takes for your neurons to fire, wire, and let new practices become habits. However, if you want to try out each change for longer and even more mindfully before you welcome in the next one, give each practice two to three days instead and complete this section in 42 to 63 days. Some of the suggested changes may already be part of your lifestyle; if that is the case, pause on those days and be even more curious about understanding their impact on your well-being.

This is also a good time to clarify the meaning behind the popular Ayurvedic belief that "one size doesn't fit all." The truth is that one size does. Warm and moist is where everyone feels most comfortable in their bodies. But most of us are off this spectrum; therefore, to return to the center, we may need slightly different tools, hence the popular Ayurvedic belief that one size doesn't fit all. It's true, but only till you find your center.

YOUR INNER CLIMATE®

Before we turn to the practices, I want you to explore your own Inner Climate®. Once you get a broad sense of where your Inner Climate® stands today, you can tweak the practices slightly to suit yourself. Use your body's intelligence to make adjustments and turn the knob up or down on what you think seems to be working to keep it warm and moist. After all, your body already knows.

The Inner Climate® Word Association Chart

HUMID	DRY	HOT	COLD	WARM & MOIST
Sticky	Anxious	Anger	Contraction	Flow
Slimy	Scatterbrained	Acidity	Shivering	Surrender
Heavy	Light-headed	Intense	Constricted	Comfortable
Phlegmy	Exhausted	Fiery	Stuck	Balanced
Mucusy	Shaky	Burning	Stubborn	Harmony
Yeast	Rough	Burnout	Cold	Fuzzy
Moldy	Noise sensitivity	Inflammation	Restrictive	Effortless
Lethargic	Weak	Inflamed	Numbing	Equilibrium
Bored	Sleeplessness	Lava	Dense	Flourishing
Stagnant	Worried	Fumes	Unstimulated	Rejuvenated
Sleepy	Windy	Hot	Dull	Thriving
Fatigue	Bloated	Heat	Inhibiting	Effortless

HUMID	DRY	HOT	COLD	WARM & MOIST
Dense	Depleted	Hot Flashes	Blocked	Nourished
Sluggish	Drained	Sharp	Frozen	Enriched
Depressed	Dry	Strong	Slowing	Peaceful
Withdrawn	Cranky	Harsh	Frigid	Vibrant
Lazy	All over the place	Impatient		Supple
Thick plaque overgrowth	Brittle	Snappy		Radiant
	Flaky	Redness		Connected
	Unsettled	Rash		Content
	Frazzled	Stressed		Adaptive
	Desiccated	Hyper-focused		Responsive
	Sparse	Control-freak		Balanced
	Disconnected	Hungry		Coherent
	Withered	Inflamed		Synchronized
		Tender		Agile
		Raw		
		Pus		

WHICH WORDS RESONATE WITH YOUR INNER CLIMATE®?

I'd like you to go through the Word Association Chart above and identify all the words you can relate strongly to.

1.　Write down your top three to five physical and mental symptoms. Are they reflected in the words you've marked out? If not, find words that describe your symptoms and mark those, too. Double-check the words to ascertain that they aptly describe the symptoms of both your body and mind. Each symptom may or may not fit more than one word from the different groupings. Or you may find yourself applying the same word to different symptoms. For example, you may have an intense rash and also experience bouts of anger, and feel raw, burning, and tender. You can mark out these words twice.

2. Which column has the most marked-out words? Humid or Dry? Hot or Cold? How many words do you have in the Warm & Moist column? Are you able to connect the dots to notice the climatic patterns of your body and mind?

3. It's common for people to have some properties of an opposing nature, so focus on those qualities that show up the most in the core of your body and mind. If you find opposing qualities in the extremities of your body (such as symptoms relating to the skin, fingertips, and toes) and in the inner core (symptoms pertaining to the digestive system and other internal organs) of your body, lay more emphasis on the words that describe the inner core.

4. Then, pay attention to the category in which you have marked the most words. Now try to picture your body as a landscape. You may realize that your body is hot and dry like a desert, hot and humid like the Amazon rainforest, or just very dense, slow, and bulky, and perhaps even cold, dry, and depleted like a cold desert. Know that this is just a start; you don't need to get it perfectly right, and your understanding will evolve and become more grounded with time. But as a preliminary exercise, this will help you to start understanding your current Inner Climate® so you can make choices that will help you to

restore the warm and moist as you move further into the book. Read the descriptions below to learn more about your possible Inner Climate®.

Humid and Cold: Your body may be over-nourished and sluggish. You may have a sedentary lifestyle; perhaps you even use food as a coping mechanism. Inherently, you are a people pleaser. You could often feel stuck in life. You may have similar thought patterns, feeling resentment, hopelessness, shame, and lethargy. It's hard for you to exercise and to keep your levels of exercise consistent, even though you have likely been told that exercise holds the key to your progress.

Dry and Cold: You are probably the queen of anxiety and may even feel very depleted. You skin may be dry, and you often feel bloated. Chances are that you don't have complete bowel movements. Scanty periods, light sleep, and worry are friends of those who are dry and cold. You know somewhere within you that you need grounding and moisture. I wouldn't be surprised if you have deprived yourself of food or another form of essential nourishment at some point in the past.

Humid and Hot: Inflammation, puffiness, and heat are at the top of your list. If you don't sweat enough, this may even feel worse and even result in skin conditions and allergies. Your periods are probably heavy and full of clots. Anger, intensity, and impatience are probably synonymous with you.

Dry and Hot: Solar is your middle name. You have likely burned yourself out with perfectionism and hard work. Your gut is probably hot and there is a chance that you have tenderness, inflammation, allergies or even an autoimmune condition. Skin conditions are not uncommon in those who are hot and dry. As you get older, your snappiness and anger become more evident, but so does the dryness on your skin and the harshness in your features. I would not be surprised if you have patches of dry eczema. But you are probably here, reading this, because you feel depleted and are seeking real change.

Now, you may not fit the exact descriptions above, but use these as a starting point and continue to stay aware of any symptoms you experience and patterns your discover about yourself. Notice where they fall in the spectrum of warm and moist. It doesn't matter what the state of your current Inner Climate® is, there is hope. I have seen more times than I can count how restoring the Inner Climate® becomes a catalyst for systemic and whole healing.

I use the Word Association Chart in my own practice quite regularly. Zarna had been referred to me by an ex-client and was suffering from rheumatoid arthritis. After studying her current condition and history, I marked out her words on the Word Association Chart: hot, burning, inflamed, redness, lava, fumes, raw, pus. Zarna explained that her joints constantly felt inflamed and she'd had oozing psoriasis for many years. There was an underlying heaviness inside; she had put on six pounds in the last year and a half, even though she was fairly active. She was also a control-freak, and in her own words she told me that she had been "losing it." She was a classic case of hot and humid.

Zarna did my 21-day healing program and really began to understand her Inner Climate®. Six months later, not only was her Inner Climate® warm and moist, but she was able to navigate her conditions and life significantly better. She once sent me a picture of a bag of spicy hot cheesy snacks and a caption that read: "I would have eaten packets of these two years ago, but now I get to eat for my Climate."

Like Zarna, I want you to live and eat so that your Inner Climate® can become more warm and moist, no matter where it stands today. If your Inner Climate® is not clear to you right now, don't worry. You can still follow the practices for 21 days as they are not only designed to bring just anyone to the center, but also allow you to sense your current climate if you tune in.

For example, if you begin to add moderate spices to your food as recommended on Day 13, but notice that they feel unreasonably hot in your gut, use that as possible evidence to conclude that you're current climate is already on the hotter side. Stay vigilant so you can really begin to connect the dots.

PREPARING FOR PRACTICE

I want you to set yourself up for success for the next 21 days. You will need more space rather than time over the next few weeks. So check for space in your life. And I'm not talking about square footage in your bedroom but in your head. Are you living with chronic stress? Are you constantly preoccupied with a world problem, work problem, parenting problem, partner problem, parent problem, or personal problem? Can you turn down the volume on other areas of your life for just 21 days so you can create some headspace?

You can and should still live your normal life and tick off all your chores on your to-do list, but I'm going to ask you to take a break from your worries of the future or the regrets about the past for the next three weeks if you want the truths of your life and body to be revealed to you. To that end, I want to suggest a headspace clean-up practice that really works for me.

FREE UP SOME HEADSPACE

I strongly recommend doing the following exercise to clear up space in your life. Although it takes about one to two hours to complete, you'll be surprised to see how much weight is lifted off you by just reassigning some headspace.

1.   Write down everything that occupies your headspace on separate note papers or sticky notes.

2.   Notice any pending tasks, the ones that absolutely need to be initiated or completed in the next 21 days, and assign two possible dates for actioning each one; for example, "Project deadline: May 24, Friday, or May 30, Friday." As you write down the dates, imagine yourself actually doing the task. Strive to get it done on the first day, but if you don't, then aim to get it done by the second instead of feeling disappointed in yourself.

3.   Now look at all those worries that can't be dealt with, like tasks which you have little or no control over. Write down each one on a separate note, set an intention to let go of them, and then release them from your headspace by placing them in an envelope and sealing it. Write "Letting Go for Now to Make Space for Bigger Change" on the envelope and stow it away or bin it. Imagine yourself surrendering these worries for the next three weeks and your heart feeling strong about it. These could be about anything – like a parent's health, the outcome of the election, or somebody else's bad behavior. You may have a different perspective on some of these issues after 21 days. But the next three weeks are your time to find yourself.

4. For all items that concern the distant future, like buying a new house or reaching Everest basecamp, put those in another envelope and, this time, write: "I know you are here, but I am taking some time to enhance my life. I will be back, even more ready for you." Keep the envelope somewhere safe. Know that living in alignment will empower you to fulfill your dreams. But for now, take this time to activate the alignment.

The second thing I would recommend is not to consume any health or wellness information for the next 21 days if at all possible (I appreciate this won't be so easy if you work in the health or fitness industry). Unfollow or pause all health and wellness-related accounts and posts on your social media. Give your body a chance to trust its own experiences, tap into the cosmic wisdom of the three core principles and let its cellular intelligence awaken. Opinions on social media may not only be inaccurate or represent another person's reality, but they may create biases that will push you back into the vicious cycle of consulting outside experts. So, for only 21 days, for less than 0.01 percent of your life (if you live to be over 80), give this a shot so you can become the expert on yourself.

Thirdly, look at your calendar. Mark out the social dinner events. Three to four events in the period of 21 days are fine, but if there are more, explore the idea of taking a rain check on them or moving dinner dates to lunch. You may even consider replacing a dinner date completely with a walk in the park or a catch-up over tea. Without scaring them away, let people in your immediate ecosystem know that you are prioritizing yourself for three weeks. You don't need to spill all the beans on your work with this book just yet, but instead, allow them to notice changes in how you are showing up. And then, when someone asks or when you feel ready, share all that you have learned so that others can benefit. But for now, the focus is on you.

Lastly, use this time to build credibility in yourself. Let go of all past scripts you may be carrying that tell you that you are incapable of making shifts. Each time we break a commitment to ourselves, we stop believing in ourselves. This doesn't mean that the struggle isn't real. It is. But I can assure you that the changes you choose to make using the insights in these pages will be more sustainable than the changes you've tried to make prescriptively in the past. Only attempt the 21 days if my work has resonated with you so far and enabled you to see yourself in a new light – not just because you've always wanted to try Ayurveda, or because your friend benefited from it, or because you love to experiment.

Treat Day 1 as though it's the first day of your new life. Let these 21 days create flow in your life, and focus more on the "why" than the "what." Focus on connection, both with yourself and with the three core principles. Start with trusting in yourself and give yourself an honest chance. If at any point you accidentally go back to your old ways, bring awareness to this and accept that it can happen to anyone. It's a normal part of growth; after all, growth happens in spurts. How you deal with these exact moments determines your journey forward. Do you shame yourself and abandon the greater plan? Do you rise above it and stay inspired? The number to count is not how many times you fall, but how many times you rise from falling. Keep on rising. Keep being inspired.

As you read about each day, you will notice that most of them are divided into four sub-sections: the Wisdom, the Prep, the Practice, and the Dilemma. The Wisdom talks about the why of the practice, the Prep tells you how to prepare for it, if necessary, and the Practice is the introduction of the actual shift or practice, while the Dilemma (or Dilemmas) will cover the challenges that may come up as you reconfigure your life.

To help you measure your changes and evolution, I have included a simple chart in Appendix 3, page 298, which you can use as a template to help you to monitor your bowels, sleep, period, moods, and weight over the three weeks.

Lastly, if you have a full-time job and are already feeling overwhelmed, feel free to slow down and take three days to practice one shift before you introduce another one, as suggested earlier. You will be surprised that most shifts are not time-consuming. However, if you are not into cooking, you may feel compelled to carve some time out as we introduce shifts in your meals. I recommend starting on a Thursday so the cooking shifts happen on the weekend, and you have more time to experiment. Like everything else, as you continue to play in the kitchen, you will see that cooking gets more accessible and more efficient.

YOUR TOOLKIT

One last thing before we start: I want to acknowledge that change is hard. This is because every time we try to change, all the versions of our younger selves that we carry within us start to feel challenged about their place in our lives. After all, we've carried them in our bodies as scripts, sensations, traumas, and memories for a long time, and even though we may finally feel ready to move on, they are not. If you've ever tried to change a long-term habit before, you'll know what I'm talking about: that uncomfortable feeling, that complete lack of inspiration, those excuses that seem real in the moment, unfamiliar bodily sensations, and the strong desire to revert to an old pattern of behavior.

Most people don't know how to cope with these sorts of inner challenges and feel unable to shed their skin to metamorphose into a butterfly, so they give up trying. That's why I want to set you up for success right now. I want you to build a toolkit to support yourself, so that you can get past any triggers and old behavior patterns that lock you in the past. This toolkit will allow you to build a life that you desire and in which you can find true flow, rather than remaining swept along in the patterns of old habits. It will also allow you to process and work on your triggers, because underneath those triggers lies your unlimited potential.

A good toolkit should have three categories:

- preventative tools

- coping tools for the moment

- repair tools

Use the lists below as an à la carte menu that you can sample from. I recommend sampling as many tools as you can from the three categories then picking the ones that are effective for you.

Preventative Tools

These are the regular practices that allow you to get out of your head and into your body so you can stay calm, inspired, and grounded. They will allow you to quickly and constantly regulate your nervous system and even alter the chemical reality inside. If you use your preventative tools wisely, you may never need to dip too much into the other two types of tools.

Here are a few of my favorite preventative tools. I suggest you try all of these and keep the ones that work for you in your toolkit. You can also use any other tools that aren't listed here but which have worked for you in the past, such as hobbies you enjoy. You want to have at least two or three preventative tools to help you regulate yourself every day.

Music

Playing classical music or soothing music in the background is known to have a calming effect on the nervous system. In fact, in Ayurveda, a whole branch of healing uses music or *ragas*. A raga is a melodic framework used in Indian classical music. It's a complex structure that governs the composition and improvisation of music within a specific scale or set of notes.

The notes are believed to create a vibrational frequency that can trigger certain neurotransmitters and enable healing. I am not surprised that there are 7 musical notes, 7 chakras and 7 endorcine glands that are responsible for releasing juices that regulate body chemistry. There are plenty of healing tracks, binaural beats, nature sounds, chants, and *bija* mantras (monosyllabic chants such as "Om") available online for free. But you can listen to any other type of music, too, as long as it inspires and soothes you.

Dance

Deep-rooted emotions are often stored in the base of the spine, especially for women. In the yoga world, this is called the base chakra. (The chakras are subtle energy points in the body.) It's also where our potential lies buried underneath our pain and trauma. Dancing is a great way to let go and let it all flow. It also allows you to disconnect from your current headspace, reset your nervous system, and return to your life afresh. My clients are often surprised when they take a dance class and see how much fun it can be, even though they may not have danced for years.

Yoga

I often joke that I lose myself when I dance and I find myself with yoga, but they both bring me to the same state of bliss. Anytime we can dissolve in the moment and lose track of space and time, healing occurs and truths are revealed. Yoga asana practice is designed not just for physical exercise but mainly to release trapped energy from the body's energy centers or chakras and reroute it through breath.

Sports

Most adults think that playing sports is a luxury, but I think of it as a self-care practice. Much like yoga and dance, sports allow you to get out of your head and into your body. And again, anytime we can get into the body, we win. So if there is a sport you enjoy playing, now is the time to get into it.

Abhyanga

As described earlier, abhyanga is the Ayurvedic practice of massaging one's body with oil before showering, for example (see page 107). While I will explain the how-to of this practice later in the book, know that touch supports the release of the happy cuddle hormone, oxytocin, and massaging soothes the nervous system. Abhyanga is a grounding practice that can help lower anxiety and promote calm.

Breathwork – Pranayama

The breath is the first telltale sign of our emotional state. When we're busy, our breath shortens; when we feel rushed, it quickens; and when we're completely relaxed, it becomes subtle and almost unnoticeable. Each inhale activates the solar aspects of our body, promoting action; while each exhale triggers the lunar aspects, bringing us back to rest. When they are balanced, the nervous system is balanced. But today, we have become too solar and stressed; and this shows in our breath, which forms a pattern of short quick inhalations when we're constantly on the go. It's a very unsafe place for the nervous system. Have you ever noticed how often we exhale in a sigh after a busy, solar-charged day? It's our body's natural way of finding balance.

Moreover, you may recall that the right and left nostrils carry distinct energies. The right nostril channels solar energy, while the left channels lunar energy. When these energies are balanced, our body achieves a perfect state of warmth and moisture. A wealth of insight and exploration can be found in understanding your breath. Various pranayama and breathwork techniques offer a straightforward, mechanical way to center your mind and body. At times, these practices can be even more powerful than therapy. As we proceed through Part 3, you'll have the opportunity to practice some of these techniques.

Meditation

Traditional meditation seeks to quiet the conscious mind and block out new stimuli, allowing deeper truths and unprocessed emotions to surface. Some techniques guide you in processing these revelations, while others focus on altering your chemical state to achieve calm and grounding.

I've mentioned earlier that when I was a teenager, my father urged me to attend a 10-day Vipassana silent meditation retreat. As a chatty, carefree girl, I had no idea what to expect. This retreat marked the first time I truly explored my inner world and witnessed the profound impact it could have on my external life. It unleashed my potential and heightened my ability to recognize and connect patterns. The transformative experience left an indelible mark on me, and I continue to practice and teach various forms of meditation today.

If the idea of meditation seems intimidating, start small – just three to five minutes can be a great beginning. If there is a particular vision of your life that you wish to fulfil, it may be useful to try a visualization technique. You might be surprised at where it takes you.

Did you wonder why breathwork, pranayama, and meditation aren't mentioned earlier on this list, even though they are probably the most talked-about and effective tools? It's because I wanted to be mindful of the fact that they aren't easily accessible to everyone. We often like to overcomplicate things and find answers that are the farthest out of reach for us. Instead, my suggestion is to start where you can. If music is easy, start there. Then try dance and maybe yoga. Or perhaps start with a sport. Meet yourself where you are, and then you will naturally move on to some of the other practices.

Coping Tools for the Moment

These next set of tools will allow you to cope while you are on the battlefield, in the middle of a triggering situation. What will you do during an intense moment when you feel an emotional rush? When you are on edge and your responses are about to become reactions? Or when your inner world feels so intense that it's on the verge of shut-down? These tools will allow you to regulate yourself in the moment, so you don't get even more caught up in a pattern of entanglement but rather begin the process of healing. These belong to the second category of tools you need in your toolkit. Try each of them when you feel triggered and notice which ones work best for you.

Humming

This is my number one tool for coping on the battlefield. I'd like you to put aside this book for a few seconds and try humming. Humming instantly extends your exhalations and puts the body in rest and recovery mode, almost like a painkiller instead of leaving you to drown in a triggering situation.

When I was 11, I hurt myself pretty badly during a sports lesson at school. The cut was deep, and I was left with a six-inch scar on my left hand. I was prescribed a drug that would shrink the scar tissue in 12 weeks. The caveat was that the drug had to be injected directly into the scar tissue with a long, thick needle – every single week. I was the kind of kid who cried hysterically at the thought of being pricked, so this painful, deep needle experience was no joke for me.

The first two shots had nurses chasing me through the hospital corridors as I tried to flee. By the third, I decided to rise to the challenge. I'm not sure when I stumbled upon humming, but at some point during my weekly prick adventures, I started humming during the insertion of the needle. Suddenly everything got better, almost like someone had infused me with a painkiller. I almost got transported to another blissful place, much like a trance.

Since then, I've used humming for all types of painful experiences and procedures, including delivering my two babies, dental work, and more. While I didn't know the science behind it at first, it always worked. More recently, I realized that humming is just as effective when I notice a trigger building up, and now I use it almost daily.

There's a reason why humming is associated with a happy state of mind. But you don't always need to be happy to hum, as it also works the other way round: Humming can make you happy. So, try humming your favorite tune next time you begin to feel that restlessness creeping up.

Grounding and Focusing on Your Breath

Let's say you are in the middle of an intense discussion, and you feel your breath racing and your cheeks turning red. You know that if this goes on a little longer, words you think you have no control over may splurge out of your mouth. What do you do? Or imagine this is Day 1 of these practices and you've barely sat down for breakfast, when your subconscious mind panics at the changes you're about to make. It starts making excuses, reminding you of all the more important things you need to do, or, perhaps, even why today is the worst day to start.

In these sorts of situations, something that works for me right away is bringing my attention to the grounding of my feet, noticing how they touch the ground, the feel of the ground, and settling into that feeling. I then bring my attention to my breath and take deliberate long and soft exhalations. This instantly allows me to disconnect from the chatter of my mind and come into my body. And then the rest is easy – because the body already knows.

The Warm Blanket

As you read the book, I want you to start imagining what a sense of being warm and moist in your heart feels like to you. It may sometimes feel like a juicy hug, or a warm and cozy blanket, or like a warm mist of gratitude that fills your heart. Whatever warm and moist feels like to you, remember that feeling so you can call upon it in times of need. I especially use this tool in uncomfortable social situations – not necessarily when I am triggered but more when I'm not able to show up fully. It instantly takes me to a natural place of ease, curiosity, and compassion.

The Warm Hug

If you have access to someone who feels safe, ask for a long hug when you feel emotionally upset. Safe human touch helps the body to release oxytocin and brings that gooey, grounded feeling, helping you to reset. In fact, a conflict resolution strategy for couples is to have difficult conversations while maintaining a loving touch. It becomes impossible for the trigger to reach its height when this tool is used.

Cool Water Wash

Sometimes, excusing yourself from the battlefield for a bathroom break to wash your face with cold water can help reset the nervous system and lower the intensity of your emotions. You can then come back to the same situation with a renewed perspective. The same is true for a shower, when possible.

Repair Tools

These are essential tools for repairing damage. You don't have to use all of these tools regularly, just as and when needed.

Journaling

I like to journal every day to repair the minor cuts and bruises caused by life. Writing everything down helps me not only to empty my headspace but to free up my thoughts and see things more clearly. I personally recommend writing two to three pages without lifting your pen – just putting down all your thoughts in the order they occur. Sometimes, my journal entries could look like this:

> It's the third day, and I still haven't been able to organize the closet. It's the most annoying task. I think Su is up. I need to warm her milk. Also, I'm so grateful for the response to yesterday's program. I was really present. Oh! I forgot to respond to Kate's email...

On other days, they could be very coherent. It doesn't matter. You never need to go back and read your journal entries; you just need to get it all out and down on paper.

Trigger Transformation Journaling

There's a particular journaling technique that helps me when I am trying to work on a particular trigger or habit that is causing me distress, and it's called trigger transformation journaling. This has been the most effective way for me to recognize old behavior patterns and introduce new ones. It has four important steps:

- **Awareness:** Notice a trigger pattern you want to break, then make a mental note to look out for it whenever there's a chance that it might come up during the course of the day. For example, you might say, "I get very worked up every time my teenage daughter talks to me." Now, start noticing each time the opportunity to get triggered arises. Notice how it feels in your body and how you respond. At the end of the day, choose three instances to write about.

- **Acceptance:** As you write about the instance, notice how it feels. Accept that the situation is hard for you and it probably touches some old wounds. After all, every trigger conceals a trauma that needs to be addressed. Accept that there will be times when you've let a trigger overpower you and perhaps even reacted in a manner you don't feel proud of.

- **Forgiveness:** Our reactions often bring shame, and shame often makes us repeat the patterns. So forgive yourself if you have reacted rather than responded to the trigger.

- **New script:** Now ask yourself how you would have responded if you were feeling courage and compassion in your heart, if your Inner Climate® were warm and moist? Feel it. How would the situation be different? Write it down briefly, imagine it and try to visualize it.

This type of journaling will help allow you to re-experience triggering events from a safe place, let their intensity lower as a result and then visualize different outcomes.

Over a period of time, you will be able to rewrite trigger scripts. Getting real and vulnerable with yourself while still creating the room for change is like self-therapy, and can be very powerful.

Sleep

When you've had a rough day, are grieving, or feel worn out from a crisis, give yourself permission to sleep. There's little that a night of deep rest can't mend. Sleep purges the nervous system, making you think and feel clearly again. I personally find that retreating to bed by 8pm at least once a month helps me recover from particularly hectic periods; it works wonders.

What makes this ritual even more special is when my daughters tuck me in. This is deeply satisfying for all of us. At the time of writing, my older daughter is in her mid-teens, while the younger is still a pre-teen, so I'm usually the one saying goodnight to them. But when I go to sleep early and our roles are reversed, they gain a sense of empowerment by learning to wind down independently, and they also learn self-care by example.

Epsom Salt Baths

Soaking in a bathtub with Epsom salt can be surprisingly relaxing on a difficult day. Epsom salt consists of magnesium sulfate and soaking in a warm tub infused with it allows the body to absorb magnesium through the skin. Magnesium plays a crucial role in the body's biochemical processes and helps to regulate the body's stress response. It's also believed that the soak can help release toxins and clean the aura.

Therapy

I'm a big advocate for therapy. It is a gift to be able to work on deep-rooted issues in a safe space with proven techniques. Therapy offers a unique opportunity to gain insights into our thoughts and behaviors, fostering personal growth and emotional healing. Moreover, therapy employs evidence-based techniques tailored to your specific needs. Whether you're dealing with anxiety, depression, trauma, or relationship problems, a therapist can provide strategies that have been scientifically proven to be effective. These techniques can help you manage symptoms, improve mental health, and enhance your overall well-being.

It's also important to recognize that therapy is a collaborative process. Finding the right therapist is key to your success. If you're open to trying therapy, consider working with a few different therapists to see whose tone and style resonates with you. Each therapist brings a unique approach; establishing a good rapport is crucial for effective treatment. This trial-and-error approach can lead to your finding a therapist who truly understands and can support you.

All these tools can be big game changers and accelerate your progress. But I don't expect you to try all of them instantly. Pick out the ones that resonate with you and try them gradually. By the end of the 21 days, your goal should be to have a strong toolkit so you can keep healing from yourself, your life and your day!

DAY 1
RESTORE YOUR RELATIONSHIP WITH MEALTIMES

The Wisdom

Healing our relationship with food is the precursor to healing everything else. Unfortunately, this cannot be done through auto-suggestion, intention, or prescription alone. It's usually a deep-seated issue, so the subconscious mind needs to get involved.

Let me explain further. Our connection with food often mirrors our inner world. Perfectionists may meticulously monitor their intake, driven by a sense of fear. Individuals struggling with self-worth may swing between over-indulgence and deprivation, punishing themselves for perceived lapses. Some may find solace in excessive consumption, using food as a means to cope with inner turmoil. Meanwhile, others harbor deep-seated fears, both of food and life itself. Some simply haven't considered the impact of their eating habits on their well-being and are equally mindless about all their life choices.

Seldom do people eat the way we are meant to eat: for nourishment, fulfillment, connection, and joy. I am amazed when I recall that our relationship with food begins at the mother's breast: connected, cozy, and safe. And it's meant to stay that way. But somewhere, as we grow, we lose connection with ourselves and, as a result, lose our sacred relationship with food. The most unfortunate part is that the more people read about the issue, the more shame it brings and the more likely it is that it will trigger further binge or control patterns.

Hence, I have developed the following practice to help my clients naturally heal their relationship with food without any need for theory and excessive mental effort. This simple practice alone will awaken your cellular intelligence and create a reverence for your food. Secrets will be revealed to you, and you will surprise yourself as you see your body effortlessly reject foods that don't serve it and invite the ones that do. The side effects of this practice include minimized digestive trouble and better tolerance of all foods.

Arjav was one of those who benefited from it. By the time he came to me, he had tried everything possible to lose weight: therapy, the keto diet, and fasting. Each one had worked for a while, but as soon as he deviated from it, his body mass came back with a vengeance. His latest experiment was with a famous appetite-suppressant weight-loss drug, but he had a strong calling to give it up and find a lasting solution.

When he was referred to me by a friend, I suggested we meet over tea before we officially started working together. Recently weaned off the weight-loss drug, he came in starving and ordered a sandwich with fries. I had barely taken a sip of my tea when I noticed that he had "inhaled" his entire meal without pausing or breathing. I knew then that no nutrition plan or advice could help him: he was addicted and, for him, food was a tool to numb something deeper.

So I offered him just this one practice that I am about to offer you. Through this, he was able to tap in to his natural appetite, subconsciously connect with different foods, his own moods, and so much more. He effortlessly became much better at coping with his feelings and, for the first time in his life, started thinking about foods beyond their taste or calories. His body didn't crave the starchy sugary foods he was used to. In his previous life, mealtimes brought self-abuse and shame with them. In his current life, each mealtime feels like therapy, an opportunity to heal from his life's baggage. Four months and a few additional changes and a new exercise regimen later, he found himself 30lbs (13kg) lighter, much healthier, happier, and certainly more connected with himself and his Inner Climate®. Not only his weight but his entire being felt transformed.

The Prep

This practice requires very little preparation, but I would suggest setting aside at least 20 minutes for each of your main meals. Avoid eating while staring at a screen or on the go, and consume at least one meal in complete solitude every day. My grandfather often said that humans run about all day to put food on the table, and it's pointless if we have no time to eat in peace! So, make sure to put a pause on your day for your meals for just these 21 days so you can give this practice a fair chance and experience its profound benefits. If you feel inclined, change or buy new tableware and switch your place at the dining table so you can create new associations in the brain.

THE PRACTICE

The practice is fairly simple and requires just three steps. First, make sure you are seated comfortably while eating.

Step 1: After each bite, put down your cutlery and place your hands on your lap till you are ready to take the next one.

Step 2: Notice the texture of your food right before you swallow.

Step 3: Make sure that you have exhaled fully every now and then in between mouthfuls. Most of us eat in short inhalations and with a tense body. As a result, the body is unable to send signals of satiety to the brain. With this brain and body disconnect, you're more likely to eat for your feelings rather than your fullness.

The Dilemma

Socializing

Keeping up the practice is challenging when you are eating with your family and even more challenging at social events. So I recommend you practice as much as you can on your own in the first few days, which will make it easier to do this when real life takes over. Don't discuss this practice with others unless they notice a difference and ask you first. As a rule, I prefer to keep health-related conversations away from the dining table as they can create unnecessary anxiety for those at different points on their journey. That being said, your consumption style will soon start to create a contagious calm at the table and have an impact on everyone around you.

Mentally rehearsing this practice beforehand will drastically improve your chances of success at social events. Accept that not every bite will be perfect, but it's realistic to expect that, with a little bit of practice, every third bite will be. So, instead of attempting to notice the texture of your food and to place your cutlery down after each mouthful, be prepared to get it right one out of three times when you are out socializing. You will find yourself making better choices organically and, as a result, minimize the regret that is often the after-effect of overconsumption at social events. As you master this practice, mindful eating will become your second nature without you having to put too much of your mind to it.

DAY 2
WARM, LIGHT BREAKFAST

Wisdom

Imagine the morning outside in nature: the grass glistening with morning dew, the cool dawn air allowing the Earth to regain its lost moisture, preparing for the new day. Birds chirp softly, gradually building their chorus with the sunrise. The first rays of sunlight spark plants into photosynthesis, reaching their peak activity at midday, before subsiding as evening arrives.

We're not so different. Just like the dew, our bodies become damp and sluggish overnight, leading to morning congestion and puffy eyes. Our joints stiffen and our digestive system is slow to awaken. A cold breakfast only adds to this dilemma and will constrict your channels, hindering the stimulation of digestive enzymes. A heavy breakfast, too, would not be effectively metabolized due to the limited fire in your gut. Thus, a warm and light breakfast is ideal: warm to ignite Agni, our digestive fire; and light to respect our limited digestive capacity at this hour.

When I looked at the diets of people who live in the blue zones, places where people organically live way longer than the average today, I wasn't surprised to see that in four of the five extensively studied zones, people ate warm, cooked breakfasts. In Okinawa, people eat miso and sweet potatoes; in Sardinia, a type of flatbread with olives; in Nicoya, Costa Rica, rice, beans, and tortillas; and in Loma Linda, California, oatmeal, and whole-grain bread.

The Prep

Take a look at the breakfast suggestions listed in Appendix 1: Menu Options and Recipes on page 255. Which ones appeal to you? Have you tried any of them before? Do you have the ingredients you need at home? You may want to ask a parent or a grandparent about the foods your ancestors ate for breakfast and see if any of those appeal to you. You can even build your own options. Just make sure they are cooked, warm, and light.

THE PRACTICE

1.　Eat a light, warm breakfast, preferably after exercising and showering. "Light" means around half or less of the quantity you usually have for lunch, and "warm" means cooked or heated.

2.　If you don't feel satiated and need more, build with quantity, not variety. It's easier to digest more of the same food rather than introduce separate food items, especially in the morning. For example, if your breakfast consists of hummus with a toasted pitta bread with drizzled olive oil, take a second helping of the same rather than supplementing with a stand-alone second dish like oatmeal.

The Dilemmas

But the world loves fruit for breakfast

Fruit for breakfast has become the new health mantra, a fad that will fade in time. Fruit in the morning hours only aggravates the dampness in the gut and slows everything down, shifting the Inner Climate® further away from warm and moist. One reason for the popularization of fruits for breakfast in recent times is the absence of other healthy alternatives, as well as the challenges of cooking fresh breakfast every day in a world that is racing for workplace productivity. And when compared to sugary processed cereals, fruits win hands down. But fruit doesn't stand a chance when the alternate option is a freshly cooked warm breakfast like porridge, a ragi malt (made with finger millet flour), or even sweet potatoes.

Anita came to me feeling hopeless about her persistent cold-like allergy. While she didn't have the itchy eyes and redness associated with allergies, her postnasal drip and congestion kept her breathing from the mouth all night long. As a result, she felt fatigued upon waking and was cranky all day. She had already been on a round of Ayurvedic herbs and tried neti (saline nasal wash). She'd found some relief, but the symptoms soon returned once the herbs were out of her system.

When I looked at her food journal, the first few lines pointed to the culprit: a "healthy" fruit smoothie (banana, frozen peaches, yogurt and ice). I did one more round of powdered herbs and replaced the smoothie with a warming malt. *Et voilà!* She could breathe again. I would love for you to try this practice during these 21 days like Anita did and see what it does for you. Notice your energy levels, your breath, and your bowel movements.

So, if you don't eat fruit in the morning, what is the best time to eat it? We will get there; just follow along.

Breakfast is supposed to be the biggest meal

If you grew up in the West, you probably grew up hearing that you should breakfast like a king. I always wondered where that theory came from. Part of it may be a conspiracy to keep factory workers for longer hours by delaying their lunch break. I then realized that a prominent nutritionist during the mid-20th century introduced this novel idea, even though it was not something that thriving cultures practiced in the past, nor something that was backed by scientific research. So "breakfast like a king" is a fairly recent idea which is not in line with the circadian rhythm, and the gastric juices aren't playing their best game either in the early morning hours.

I'm not hungry enough for breakfast

It's not a problem if you aren't hungry enough for breakfast. Perhaps your digestive juices and acids need a little more time to perform. In that case, stay away from breakfast but get that fire inside started with a small warm beverage, like a cup of hot spiced milk with almonds on the side.

I have no time to make a warm breakfast

Stress not; instead, just throw some sourdough in the toaster and drizzle a little olive oil on it when it's done. Sourdough bread is the only type of bread I would ever recommend since it's made using a natural fermentation process that supports our warm and moist Inner Climate® and also gives rise to *Lactobacillus reuteri*. This is the same strain of bacteria that is found in breastmilk, and that actively helps establish a healthy gut microbiome and develop immunity in babies.[4] There is no other food that carries this strain. So you basically get some of the advantages of breastmilk but through your bread. Is that not music to your ears?

Also, sourdough bread has a lower glycemic index than other breads and will not cause your blood sugar levels to spike. Not only that, the lactic acid bacteria support the breakdown of gluten, making it OK even for those who are gluten-sensitive. My only ask is that you source high quality, fresh sourdough from a local bakery whenever possible.

DAY 3
HEAVY LUNCH, EARLIER DINNER

The Wisdom

Even though the body can adjust to a degree to whatever routine you put into place, you already know the endless benefits of following the circadian rhythm. Ideally, the exogenous clock should trump your endogenous clock. In simple words, you let the rhythms of the universe design your day rather than working against the tide of your juices to create your personal body clock.

It's time to start putting this into practice now. If there is just one thing you take away from the book, let this one be it. The Agni, the body's metabolic ability, is activated at sunrise and naturally peaks midday before it dwindles with sunset. It makes sense for our food patterns to follow the same order so we can take advantage of what I call "the Agni supporters."

The first Agni supporter is gastrin, which is released in the stomach to regulate gastric juices, gastric motility or movement, and which is active during digestion. It also regulates gastric mucosal growth, the protective lining inside the digestive tract. While gastrin is released in response to food, studies show that gastrin, according to its circadian behavior, naturally peaks between the hours of 10am and

2pm, and then gradually declines.[5] Naturally, you want to eat when your internal stove is cooking at its best.

The second Agni supporter is ghrelin, the hunger hormone. Ghrelin production starts in the morning and rises through the day. It is produced in the stomach and travels through the blood to the brain, pestering it to look for food when the levels are sufficient. The longer we let ghrelin rise, the more ravenous our hungry hormone becomes, compelling us to look for energy-dense foods. This means that if we were to eat light during the day and let dinner be our day's main event, we would be working with really high ghrelin levels that need starchy, heavy foods to let leptin, the satiety hormone, come in and say, "Stop!" This is counter-productive, as our third Agni supporter, insulin, is the weakest at night.

Insulin, the blood-sugar-regulating hormone produced by the pancreas, is released when the body needs to break down sugar. However, the body is more sensitive to insulin during the daytime and resistant to it during the evening and night hours. Simply put, blood sugar can be regulated more easily during the day, specifically around midday.

The behavior of all three "Agni supporters" is evidence that our digestion does best at lunchtime, which is ideal for our biggest meal. It takes a little getting used to, but you'll notice the difference in your sleep, bowels, and skin immediately.

Once again, nighttime means lowered gastrin levels and increased insulin resistance, making it the perfect time to forego eating and fall into what nature intended to be a natural form of intermittent fasting. I would also like to mention that eating late increases the possibility of you sleeping with undigested food in your stomach. Instead of the body going into deep repair, it now has to work to break down whatever it can do, so toxic waste doesn't accumulate in your system.

The Prep

As prep for the next few practices, I would suggest you bring cooking into your life. While it may sound like a chore, getting into the kitchen, when possible, can be very grounding and meditative. Engaging all your senses, touching your foods, and seeing them transform is an intimate experience that allows you to begin restoring your relationship with meals. However, when you cannot cook, it may be better to order fresh food from a restaurant with a quick turnaround rather than eating leftovers. But more on that in the coming days.

For now, you want to start collecting plenty of quick lunch and dinner recipes. Most people in the West don't make it home in time to be able to cook an early dinner. So prep for dinner before you leave home, use an electric slow cooker or rice cooker, and set a timer if you can so your meal will be ready quickly upon your arrival home. Feel free to use the recipes and menu ideas provided on pages 255–93 or to experiment on your own.

THE PRACTICE

1. Make lunch the most substantial meal of the day. Use your peaking gastric juices to consume anything you've been dreaming of. Remember that lunch is the most forgiving part of the day when it comes to your digestive system.

2. Finish eating dinner before 6.30pm or 7pm so your body doesn't have to work during its downtime. You can probably relate to the inefficiency that comes with extra-long hours of work, and our digestive system is no different.

The Dilemmas

Late-night hunger

If you are used to eating later at night, let me warn you right now that the first three days of change are going to be the hardest. Your endogenous clock (the one that gets used to your behavior) is going to be unhappy about it. It likes its habit of eating later, so brace yourself for its reaction.

If you feel uncontrollable hunger a few hours after your early dinner, drink a hot cup of milk spiced with cardamom. If milk is not your thing, chew on a few roasted almonds with a cup of chamomile tea. Remember, this too shall pass; before you know it, your body will embrace this alignment.

But I feel sleepy after lunch...

It's not uncommon to feel a slump after eating lunch. But this is especially true if you've had a big or a cold breakfast earlier that morning and your Agni was never fully kindled to its full midday capacity. But it can happen due to other reasons as well, like the changing seasons, a really early morning rise, foods rich in carbohydrates, or overeating during lunch. That being said, a slight lethargy is natural for almost everyone as our blood rushes to the digestive system and away from the brain after a meal.

Ayurveda recommends walking about 100 to 200 steps after eating and lying on your left side with your head propped up against your hand, like the laying-down statue of Buddha, for about 15 to 20 minutes where possible. This will not only begin to support the descent of your food through your digestive system, but it will activate the left side of the body, which is associated with building heat and thus activating digestion.

Eating out

I've been unable to wrap my head around the concept of late-night dinner events. If I need to meet a friend after hours, it's usually for a cup of chamomile tea or a foot massage. But I understand that it's not always in your hands, so if you do find yourself at a dinner event, I recommend you eat a light supper at home first. This way, your levels of ghrelin, the hunger hormone, won't be soaring when you're out, and you won't have the urge to overindulge. Instead of trying everything on the menu, focus on one main item and eat a small amount, remembering to put your cutlery down in between mouthfuls.

Eating with the seasons

The one question I always get asked is, "How do we shift our dinner times according to the seasons?" After all, the sun can set as early as 3pm in the winter for a lot of earthlings. The simple answer is you still eat dinner around your usual time. If changing it at all, you may move your dinner by 30 to 60 minutes to an earlier time in the winter and push it back by the same amount of time in the summer. But you want your body to follow your endogenous clock (the behavior your body is used to, versus the external circadian cues) during these seasonal shifts if you live in a region where the length of the day varies significantly from summer to winter.

DAY 4
LIGHTER DINNER

The Wisdom

My ask today, on Day 4, is that you eat a lighter meal in the evening, and it's an extension of Day 3's practice, as your gut's inner army is at its weakest at this hour. Right here, I'm going to raise my expectations of you, but with the promise that in return, your nights will be transformed. You will feel lighter, experience overall better digestion and sleep; and once you learn to cope with the crankiness that may arise with not using food as a coping mechanism after hours, you will even notice more clarity of thought and even a natural desire to introspect.

Not burdening the body with digestion at night means that you experience benefits similar to fasting, not only at a physical level but also a spiritual level. Fasting usually allows the body to breakdown any excesses, but fasting at night additionally supports the cleanup of debris in the nervous system that gets accumulated due to thinking. When you stop feeding the material body more material, energy is released. In Ayurveda, we call this a *Sattvik* state of mind, the state of mind that allowed the yogis to cut through the chatter of the conscious mind and dive into their subconscious.

Another major factor is that most people are tired and stressed out by the time evening arrives, so it's natural for the mind to switch off and indulge in mindless eating. This practice eliminates that possibility.

Eating light and early is also extremely important if you're looking to be at your optimum weight. One of the main risk factors for obesity in night-shift workers is the consumption of large meals, late at night.

The Prep

Keep herbal teas, almonds, or milk to hand, just in case you absolutely cannot resist your oral addiction and want to consume something after your early and light dinner. Once again, be prepared that the first three days will feel the most challenging.

THE PRACTICE

Reduce the quantity of your dinner to 50 to 60 percent that of lunch. Know that your body is ready to do only half the work digestively, so give it half the food.

I personally like to consume a bowl of soup with a side of something small like stir-fried veggies or even a little helping of a rice dish. Once again, refer to Appendix 1 on page 255 for meal ideas and more.

The Dilemmas

Dinner is family time

If dinner is the only time your family comes together around a table, and not eating dinner with the family feels blasphemous, I hear you. But you could start a health trend in your family and inspire others, reducing everyone's risk for obesity, diabetes, and other conditions related to eating heavy dinners.

Priya had found me as a result of her quest to try the next health fad. A 33-year-old from India, she had consulted various other experts and gotten on and off several trends. Until now, she'd fundamentally believed that achieving good health required a secret code that couldn't be found on your own. When she saw her thyroid levels and the reading on her weighing scales lower to more desirable levels with what she called "intuitive ancient wisdom," she was surprised. After her initial disbelief, she was sold. A year later, she was looking to pursue a career in the field of sustainable health.

Life was working out for her and she even got married to the man of her dreams. This is when the dilemma presented itself. Her husband lived with his parents and his extended family, as is often the case in traditional Indian families. They loved her and she reciprocated, but they often expressed how unhappy they were with her choice of not eating 9pm dinners with the family. Priya felt frustrated but lovingly stood her ground and sat with her cup of herbal tea every night as the rest of the family dined.

Family planning was next on the cards and as suggested by her doctor, the couple got thoroughly tested to see where they stood with their fertility. While Priya passed with flying colors, her husband's reports showed issues with sperm motility, the ability of the sperm to swim. The doctors' first ask was that he lose the extra pounds his body carried. Priya was able to work with her husband to achieve his goal and one of the primary changes he made was to join his wife in having light and early dinners. On my last trip to India, I found out that not only was Priya pregnant, but that her entire family was now eating dinner at 7pm and as a result felt much healthier and more energetic. They'd had the chance to witness the transformation light and early dinners had brought about and naturally followed suit.

I'm not saying that you should expect the same shift in your ecosystem but chances are that over time, you will inspire someone. The caveat is that you mustn't impose, nor should you give unsolicited advice. If someone becomes curious about it, let them know how the practice supports you, rather than advocating that they try it too.

Another important part is to show up at the dinner table completely relaxed with your cup of herbal tea. This way you are more present and fun and no one will have to miss out on your company, nor are they put out by your resistance to conform.

I'm bored ...

As the day loses its shine, dinner is what many look forward to. Without a heavy dinner, evening boredom and anxiety can set in, especially if dinner is your main event for the late evening hours. If that is the case, you want to ensure that you have something else to look forward to during this time. My personal go-to is a loving evening routine but you may also consider taking up a hobby like reading, journaling, a jigsaw puzzle, or mandala coloring. A walk in nature and classical music can also feel very grounding and help calm the nervous system. (I'll offer some suggestions for a helpful evening routine as we continue to progress through the days.)

But my cravings are strongest at night

If you experience strong cravings at night, you're not the only one. I am going to give you a simple method to deal with your cravings without actually going into deprivation. In deprivation mode, the brain experiences the threat of scarcity and as a result, you are more likely to binge later. Eventually the binge will bring shame, which may lead you to punish yourself though deprivation, once again. I want you to stay away from this deprivation–binge–shame cycle.

The solution is "Fantasize, Don't Deprive." If you spot a large piece of chocolate cake in the refrigerator at 8pm, replace the dialogue in your head. Instead of "I can't eat it, I shouldn't eat, I am not supposed to eat it but I really want it," tell yourself, "This decadent cake is so inviting and I will eat it at lunch tomorrow. I am going to relish each bite when I do." This simple shift in your self-talk can trigger a significantly different response in your brain chemistry and thus your actions. Instead of the hopelessness that comes with deprivation, it allows you to build hope, and feel less insecure by just delaying gratification. When tomorrow arrives, you can enjoy that cake as fantasized, during the daytime. However, there's a chance that you'll have moved on and no longer desire the cake at all. And if you do choose to eat it, your body will now be more prepared to receive it!

NO COLD BEVERAGES

The Wisdom

If you live in the Western part of the world, your gullet is probably used to cold fluids, but you probably know too well by now that cold liquids can be a like a snowstorm in your tropical gut, destroying life there slowly. It may be helpful to revisit the chapter "The Gut and Your Diet" in Part 2 to refresh your memory even further.

By its very nature, cold simultaneously constricts and contracts; thus, cold water shrinks the diameter of microscopic body channels, and cannot travel far and wide. However, a warmer beverage expands everything and goes down sip by sip. It waters the body lovingly, just as we would water our plants, not by dunking them in water all at once, but gradually, for optimum absorption.

Warmer water may not feel as satisfying at first, but within a few weeks, you will see your overall need for water go down and your body will feel more hydrated.

I recommend adding herbs to your water, too, either to suit the season or to support your current Inner Climate®. This will make your warm water tastier, as well as giving it richer health-giving properties.

The Prep

Fill a 16fl oz. (approx. 500ml) thermos flask with hot water. Choose from the options below to add to your water. The quantity of the herb is not important, but start with one heaped teaspoon of dried herbs or a handful of fresh herbs. Steep for 2–5 minutes and strain out or let them float if you prefer instead. Increase or decrease the amount based on personal preference.

HERBS	WHEN TO USE
Mint	Summer or if nauseous
Licorice	Inflammation
Carom seeds	Winter or if you have a cold or are bloated
Cumin	On days your tummy feels sensitive
Chamomile flowers	Second half of day or when sick

If there is another herb that you know works for you, go for it. If you aren't averse to the taste, I would recommend adding a pinch or two of dried organic ginger to this water. Dried ginger is known to stabilize Agni. Both TCM and Ayurveda worship dried ginger. Wait for the water to cool down to a warm temperature before you pop the lid back on.

THE PRACTICE

Drink this water, one sip at a time, throughout the day. If warm water makes you uncomfortable, you may wish to wait till it becomes room temperature by simply pouring it into a cup. When you finish the first thermos, fill the flask again with water. You don't need to replace the herbs. Drink according to how thirsty you are, even though you may just realize that you are naturally more satiated and feel less thirsty unless it's a really hot day.

Try to finish 80 percent of your water intake between the hours of 10am to 4pm. Drinking water after sunset usually means a damper gut and more trips to the bathroom in the middle of the night.

If you go to a restaurant, make sure to ask them for hot water or, at the very least, water without ice. Make herbal teas your beverage of choice as much as possible, so you can metabolize your foods better. After all, you are giving this practice a fair chance for 21 days.

The Dilemmas

Smoothies

Your cold consumption for the day may just be a glass of smoothie. If you have bought into the smoothies fad, and have successfully used them to lower your appetite and feel mentally great about yourself, this is for you.

Yes, cold smoothies will temporarily shut down gut activity and slow things down inside, interrupting all life like a snowstorm would, and making you feel less hungry as a result. You may end up consuming fewer calories and feel great, as we are trained to believe that lighter calories mean more health.

But in the long term, cold smoothies will systematically alter the environment of the gut and spiral into other imbalances. This doesn't mean that you should never have smoothies; feel free to indulge occasionally on a warm day when the sun is still out.

However, replace smoothies with fresh fruit and even Ayurvedic buttermilk (see page 280) when possible. And if you are concerned about the intake of superfoods that you regularly add to your smoothies, don't worry. Once you start eating Ayurvedically, these superfoods will organically make it into your meals. No extra effort is required.

But my body craves cold beverages

If you find yourself regularly craving cold beverages, it's likely your gut has trapped heat that your body is struggling to dissipate and regulate. This trapped heat drives your constant desire for cold fluids. However, relying on cold drinks for relief isn't a sustainable solution. While it might provide temporary comfort, it can actually destabilize your Agni (digestive fire), making it even more erratic and potentially worsening the issue.

Another common reason for craving water, particularly after meals, is overeating. When you overeat, your gut heats up like a bustling kitchen, working overtime to kick-start the metabolic processes. Additionally, consuming extremely hot, spicy, acidic, sour, or processed foods can also fuel this internal heat, prompting your body to seek out cold water to cool down the digestive system.

RE-EVALUATE YOUR RELATIONSHIP WITH SCREENS

The Wisdom

I wish we could all merely set an intention to repair our relationship with our screens and it would just happen, but I know that this one is even trickier than changing our habits with food. I've struggled with it, too. Firstly, it is far more pervasive since they are easily accessible to us 24/7. Secondly, the ill effects aren't noticeable in the short term, so the tendency to indulge is greater. Thus, repairing this habit requires more checks and balances.

I remember when cable television first came about, I disliked the idea of channel surfing. I was able to tune in to the unease and anxiety it caused to my nervous system and thus managed to avoid it altogether. While the same discomfort arises when we scroll mindlessly on our phones, it has become so habitual that we've made it the new normal. Most of us don't even know the possibilities that life can present without cellphones. How much more present we would be? How much more deeply immersed in each moment? Some of my biggest breakthroughs have happened on long Wi-Fi-free flights from or to India.

Cellphone browsing is a solar activity, not only because of the rapid activity it brings to the nervous system but also because of blue-light exposure. I am not surprised that cellphone usage has increasingly been linked to anxiety and other mental health conditions.

Well, if you are feeling withdrawal symptoms already, let me assure you that I am not asking that you give up your cellphone completely but that you regulate its usage in the evening hours and see what happens to your time and presence as a result.

The Prep

As prep for this one, I would like you to explore more of yourself rather than your social media feed at the end of the day. The time that would normally be dedicated to mindless and endless scrolling is now going to be dedicated to you. It's your bonus time at the day's descent. What interest might you explore tonight? Prepare for it ahead of this practice. Feel free to borrow from ideas that were suggested on Day 3: journaling, mandala coloring, etc. Get a journal ready, or perhaps print out some mandalas that you can color in. If you like to read, make sure you have a good book waiting by your bedside.

THE PRACTICE

Put your phone on airplane mode 60 minutes before bedtime, or leave it out of the room if you choose to keep it switched on. Let your closest ones know that you will generally not be available at nighttime and finish your day's closing messages before you set aside your phone.

Use this time for yourself instead. This is your time, take it. Even if this means that it brings complete boredom. Boredom is often an entry point to something more meaningful. So enjoy simply sitting with yourself. This simple practice can be an absolute game changer, allowing you time for introspection.

The Dilemmas

Addiction to your cellphone

The experiences of the day can touch certain nerves and bring about certain feelings. While we can bring more awareness to them, it is virtually impossible for us to process these feelings every single time that they occur. As a result, the discomfort from the feelings gets stored in the body. Evenings can feel particularly uncomfortable because of the day's accumulated baggage. What makes it worse is that daytime excitatory mediators, the juices that keep us excited, are naturally subdued to make room for the inhibitory mediators, which help you prepare for shut-down. According to Ayurveda, the state of the body is rapidly changing during this transition and this can bring with it anxiety and unease.

For both reasons, it's common for people unconsciously to reach out for numbing mechanisms by the time evening arrives. While alcohol and food are the often talked about as being coping vices, cellphone browsing is not much different. So if a screen has become your way to unwind at the end of a loaded day, I get you. But I want you to remember that when the sun is down, these last hours of the day open up a portal to the self, so you want to connect with this instead of numbing it.

While journaling is my favorite way to connect with myself, you can connect through anything that grounds you.

When your body is immersed in an activity for the sake of the activity and not obsessed with the outcome, you will lose a sense of time and space. And when you dissolve in this manner, healing begins and boundless possibilities open up.

Insecurity

We are so used to being accessible via our cellphones that going off the grid can bring about a tremendous fear of missing out. *What if someone needs me? What if something bad happens and someone tries to reach me?* I don't blame you for this. In this world, where a lot of us live far away from our loved ones, we find greater security in being easily contactable.

But that being said, what was the last time someone tried to reach you in the middle of the night for an emergency or crisis? In the course of our lifetime, we may get one or two such calls at the most. But even then, how many times can we change an outcome that was meant to be?

When my grandfather was on his deathbed in India, my family tried to reach me in New York. I was standing in the rain, queuing on the street for an unimportant sample sale. My ringtone volume couldn't compete with the traffic orchestra of NYC. Even though it was the middle of the day and my cellphone was on me, I missed that call and regretted it. And yet the outcome for him was unchanged.

Another time, I woke up to see 11 missed calls from different members of my family. I panicked. I called another relative and asked him to come over before I could return the calls. I held his hand and prayed as he dialed. The news was that my cousin had just delivered a baby girl. Phew! I was relieved. But I would have been just as thrilled in the morning, perhaps even more so. The outcome, once again, was unchanged.

So let your loved ones know that you're going off the grid every night. And if that still brings discomfort, leave your phone outside the room set at an audible volume.

NO SHOWERING OR EXERCISING WITH FOOD IN YOUR STOMACH

The Wisdom

Confession: There are days when I cheat and consume cold beverages, especially if I'm out on a hot and humid day; at other times, I may even indulge in a late-night pizza with my girls, but breaking the rule of not showering or exercising with food in your stomach is sacrilegious and one we never ever bend. Every time you eat and go into the shower after eating, the heat that was building up in your gut gets rerouted to your extremities as your body begins to thermoregulate. Any food that was in its mid-digestion phase is now unattended and left to rot and ferment in your warm insides. Ayurveda compares this undigested food to slow-acting poison and calls it Ama. This Ama can then travel through the body's channels, affecting energy levels, immune function, and the overall Inner Climate®. It's like land that's covered in marsh. And I know that's not what you want; you are aiming for warm, moist, and lush.

Exercising with food in the stomach is not very different. Exercise can be intense for the body, and certain types of exercise, like walking or running, can direct heat to the limbs and other parts. Once again, the gut is distracted, and digestion is aborted, leading to the formation of Ama. You may argue that your exercise is focused on the gut and should thus help digestion, but that isn't true. When exercise builds heat in the body and your body begins to sweat, the gut can become excessively hot, much like a hot kitchen with no ventilation. It's not uncommon for people who exercise after eating to experience acidity, migraines, and burning. This can also lead to skin conditions like eczema in the long term.

So, if you want to keep the climatic condition in your gut conducive to healthy digestion and nutrient absorption, and to get the best from the great food choices I know you will make, remember that the order of consumption is paramount.

The Prep

Plan your day and mind well in advance so you can stick to the new proposed order of events.

THE PRACTICE

Avoid exercising or showering with food in your gut at all costs. Instead, start thinking about a morning routine where you have time to shower and exercise before you eat. Both these activities stimulate the damp morning gut, kindle Agni, and will make your breakfast more satisfying and easy to digest. This one is certainly a no-brainer.

Dilemmas

I feel hungry in the morning

If you wake up famished, your gastric juices are acting up before their time. But as you rewire your life, you will be able to wake up without the urgent need to eat. For now, satisfy yourself with half a cup of hot milk diluted with half a cup of hot water and boiled together with some cardamom or another spice. Alternatively, you can chew on a few soaked and peeled almonds. Wait 20 to 30 minutes before you start exercising.

I can't exercise on an empty stomach

Once again, you probably have excess acid in your gut that makes you prematurely hungry or you may be running on low glucose levels. There are a few things that may work for you, depending on where the issue stems from. (Abhyanga or oil massage is essentially food for the body before exercise, but more on that later, on page 201.) You can also try chewing a couple of dates. Dates are a very special food because they instantly give you the feeling of satiety without adding bulk to your stomach. If that's impossible, eat breakfast first but wait for a while before you exercise and shower.

How long should we wait to shower or exercise after eating?

If you haven't yet been able to design a day where you can exercise and shower in the morning before breakfast, you may be asking this question. The time you should wait to shower and exercise after eating will depend entirely on the quantity of the meal and the rate at which you digest your food. As a rule of thumb, wait an hour at least after a light breakfast or two hours after a moderate lunch, or even a light dinner. But what's even more important is that you shouldn't be able to feel any trace of the meal sitting in your gut.

EXERCISE

The Wisdom

There is no substitute for exercise. An active lifestyle and walking back and forth from work or college don't count. Exercise is a systematic, planned activity that allows your body to move in ways that it otherwise would not. It allows your body to sweat and breaks down excess tissue, releases toxins, stimulates organs, strengthens tissue and the heart, moves and lubricates the joints, warms up the gut, and builds an appetite – provided you do it right.

Let's recall the two exercise rules in Part 2. Firstly, exercise to half your capacity and stop when you become breathless and break into a sweat. Secondly, good fats should be consumed during mealtimes on those days you are exercising to prevent the depletion of soft essential tissues in the body. Moreover, the morning hours between 6am and 10am are the best time to exercise to offset the naturally present dampness.

You want to choose your form of exercise according to your Inner Climate®. For example, if your climate is sluggish, humid, and dense, you need exercise that makes you sweat and loosens you up, like spinning or dancing. Once your insides have gotten moving, add a form of exercise that builds strength, like Pilates, yoga, or swimming. Once you feel strong in your joints, you can introduce slightly more intensive forms of training.

If you're depleted and dry, be careful how much you exercise and what form you choose. Hot yoga, functional training, and high-intensity training may dehydrate your juices and harden your tissues. Restorative yoga, Pilates, and walks in nature are your thing. Once you've nourished yourself with warm and moist foods like sweet potatoes with ghee or avocados on fresh sourdough with a drizzle of olive oil and spices, you will see that over a period of time, your body will feel more nourished, your skin will be moister and your mind will become less anxious. Feel free to become a little more adventurous with your exercise then.

For those with hot and humid Inner Climates®, feeling puffy and inflamed regularly, you want to be mindful of this. If your body sweats easily upon exercise, it's a good sign. It shows that your body's mechanism for cooling down is in place. And yet you want to be careful not to dehydrate yourself too much. Stay away from hot yoga, high-intensity training, and anything that overheats your system. For you, swimming, yoga, Pilates, nature walks, dance, and low-intensity spin classes could work. On days that you are feeling particularly solar, go for a nature walk if the day is cool. Drinking coconut water 30 minutes after your workout could be a game changer.

But if you're hot and dry and unable to sweat, you have more to think about. Your body may lack the fluids it needs to sweat, or your fluids have become hot and thick, like lava trapped inside. Your body may be unable to thermoregulate and cool down effectively. Acupuncture and cupping treatments could get things moving. An Ayurvedic treatment called bloodletting could also get things flowing. Either way, low-intensity yoga, walking in the moonlight, and swimming would be forms of exercise that I'd recommend.

My personal favorite forms of exercise are yoga, dance, spin class, and a long walk in Central Park here in NYC. Occasionally, I like to take a Pilates or a stretch class, too.

Prep

Set your morning alarm to a time 40 minutes earlier than you would otherwise, so you increase your total waking hours by the same amount of time that I am asking you to exercise for. What will your exercise be? Plan for it. If you haven't exercised for a while, be prepared for some possible inertia to set in. What tool are you going to use to get past that?

THE PRACTICE

Exercise for 40 minutes on six out of seven days a week. Take one day off for rest and recovery.

Instead of just mindlessly exercising, think about your Inner Climate® and what your body and mind need for the day.

Make sure you have included more than one form of exercise each week.

The Dilemmas

I have no time in the morning

My first recommendation would be to make the time for exercise by getting up earlier. But if that's impossible, try to get your exercise done before 11am. If evening is the only time you can exercise, the only exercise forms I would recommend are walking outside in nature and restorative yoga. Evening exercise can excite and wake up the system instead of winding it down. Yes, it will tire your muscles, and you may even sleep well, but your body will choose to work more on recovery from the exercise rather than the deep cellular repair that happens every night.

I feel very lazy

If you haven't exercised for a while, your struggle is understandable. But the more you think about it, the harder it will become. Instead, imagine how your body feels when you move and try fantasizing about the after-effects, rather than treating exercise like obeying a strict order. Choose an exercise form that you like.

Valerie had accepted that exercise wasn't her thing, yet every now and then she secretly wished she could get her body moving. Each time she did, it lasted only for a few days. Once people started noticing her chisel and muscle-tone, the self-sabotage began. Her mind started playing games on her, and she found a reason to stop. After years of this pattern, she didn't even want to try.

But that isn't why she came to me; she came to me for help with her depression. I knew that depression makes the body even more stagnant, and that further perpetuates the problem; it becomes a vicious circle. So, exercise was a non-negotiable. Given her love for music, I encouraged her to pick a dance fitness class, and we made a deal that she had to stay only for three songs and could then leave the class if she desired. The caveat was that if she decided to stay for the fourth song, she had to stay for another three in total, and then if she stayed for six songs and wanted to stay for the seventh one, she had to stay for a total of three more. So, staying for any additional song meant staying for an increment of three. I also asked her to throw out her old exercise wear and buy new bright and sexy clothes.

We agreed that she wouldn't talk about what she was doing too much to others, and every time her mind started chattering about the planning or hardship of exercise, she was to try to bring her attention to her body or breath. Our last deal was that she couldn't consume sugar until she finished her exercise for the day. Even with the rules around it, this felt like low pressure to her. "Three songs can't be that bad; I don't have an instructor monitoring my reps, I can adjust my intensity, I get to eat sugar, and I have to do this only three times a week," she thought.

What do you think happened? The first dance class was hard. She stood at the back, looking around, and moved her body slowly for three songs. By the third class, she felt more comfortable; by the seventh class, she stayed for six songs. After a year, she was contemplating becoming a fitness dance instructor herself. She later told me that she had always thought of exercise as punishment and had chosen really hard routines the few times she got into it. As a result, it was not enjoyable or sustainable.

The key is to pick something you'll enjoy and start small, really small. Don't talk about it too much to others; know that your mind will chatter, and you need to return to your body to create a sense of warm safety and keep going. Give yourself possible exit points to lower the pressure, but have rules around them, like staying for three songs at a time, 20-minute slots in a spin class, and 10-minute increments in a yoga class. I always prefer to measure the length of my routine in terms of music tracks rather than time. Music and exercise are buddies. Just start and build, slowly and sexily. Enjoy your body and its ability to move and heal.

I have been exercising, but my weight doesn't budge

Yes, this can happen, especially if you have dense tissue that hasn't received exercise for a while. I want you to think of dense fat tissue as being like tightly packed glue molecules. They need a lot of heat before they start to melt. It's also like cold milk that takes a while to boil. Make sure you choose exercise that makes you sweat. In my experience, the magic number is three weeks of consistent exercise; that's when things start to move, even for those who have previously been immobile. At the same time, don't let exercise become an excuse to overeat. Stick with the other practices in the 21 days and see the difference.

PLAY WITH YOUR CAFFEINE INTAKE

The Wisdom

Caffeine is hot and drying (dehydrating); no wonder it stimulates us and keeps us focused, before it burns us out to a point of depletion and keeps us asking for more. If your body is already inflamed or hot, excess caffeine will smoke your insides. If your body is dry and depleted, it will suck your succulence even further. However, if your body is gooey with plaque and cholesterol, caffeine in moderation could scrape and dehydrate some excesses. No wonder that in some parts of the world, marketers of tea call it good for the heart. They forget to add, "If your heart has cholesterol-rich blood flowing through it."

Don't get me wrong, I love my cup of chai. The idea is to play with our caffeine so it's less harmful. Firstly, consuming caffeine earlier in the day when the environment is still wet will help. Caffeine after 3pm is too hot and dry for the system; it may aggravate and overstimulate the nervous system when it's really ready to unwind. It may even give you an illusion of extra energy while your insides are already depleted from the day's work. But even if you are consuming coffee at an earlier time, cooling and moist additions like milk, ghee, cream, cane sugar, or even a cardamom pod can help soften its blow.

There's a reason why "bullet coffee," coffee blended with ghee or butter, is now so popular.

For me, caffeine usually comes in the form of a little cup of chai, which I especially indulge in when I have company. Occasionally, I will get myself a single-shot cappuccino. But every time I go through a phase of consuming no caffeine, my energy levels and mood drastically begin to improve after the initial two to three withdrawal days.

The Prep

If you're a caffeine drinker, you can buy some milk, ghee or coconut oil to go in your beverage. You can even buy some cardamom pods as a bonus.

THE PRACTICE

My ask of you on Day 9 is a big one:

- No caffeine consumption after 3pm.

- Reduce your caffeine intake by half. If your coffee has two shots, make it one. If you drink two cups of tea, make it either one cup or two half-cups.

- Consider adding a dash of milk or blending in a teaspoon of ghee or coconut oil in your drink.

The Dilemmas

Cold caffeine beverages

If caffeine is hot and dry, does it mean that drinking iced coffee could help mitigate the ill effects of caffeine? No, the experience that it brings to your body remains unchanged. Caffeine stimulates and is inherently solar. In Ayurveda, this inherent property is called potency and most substances can be either cooling or warming; caffeine is warm in its potency. Additionally, as explained earlier in Part 3, I want you to give warm beverages a fair chance for these 21 days and see if this is something you want to bring into your life in the long term. So drink your coffee or tea warm.

Tea or coffee? Green or black tea?

All caffeinated teas come from the same plant, *Camellia sinensis*. How they are processed changes their color and potency. White tea has the least amount of caffeine and can even be enjoyed occasionally without cooler add-ons such as milk. Next is green tea, with black tea leading in the caffeine-count category. Coffee is even more potent than black tea, with significantly more caffeine.

The chart below provides a general estimate of the caffeine content in different beverages, as this can vary depending on the brand of drink, brewing or steeping time, and other factors.

Beverage	Caffeine content (per cup)
White tea	15–30mg
Green tea	30–50mg
Black tea	40–70mg
Chai (masala tea)	50–70mg
Coffee	95–200mg

Decaf drinks

Decaf coffee and tea are processed in a manner that strips away most of the caffeine, but these beverages can be ultra-processed. So, if you want to try decaf caffeine, make sure it's a specialty brand that uses more natural methods of processing.

Ideally, caffeine should be consumed between 10am and 3pm. That said, while consuming caffeine later in the day will overstimulate your nervous system, when consumed in the morning, it could overstimulate your gastric juices, affecting the body's ability to regulate Agni throughout the day.

DAY 10
SLEEP BEFORE 10PM

The Wisdom

There is no healing like the healing that happens when we are asleep. If there is one point I hope I've driven home so far, it's the importance of following the circadian rhythms, especially during the first part of the solar phase and the first part of the lunar phase. If you get your mornings right, you will get your day right. By the same token, if you get your bedtime right, you will probably get your night right.

Most people in the busy urban world wait till they're ready to drop dead from exhaustion before they hit that sack. While falling asleep at that point is easier, it's harder to remain asleep or even sleep deep for too long, as the body is depleted of the sleep hormone melatonin by then. The irony is that when we sleep at the sweet point of the body and mind being slightly unwound but not too tired, we can sleep the deepest and the longest.

Moreover, it's important for the body to go through all the phases of sleep: rest, repair, and rebuilding. When we stay up at night, we end up exhausting the energy reserves that would have been allocated to vital sleep-time repair. We also fail to replenish our bodies with the subtle moisture that nighttime sleep facilitates. Over a period of time, it can dry out our Inner Climate® and even lead to agitation and anxiety. Moreover, sleeping late can often mean waking up late and starting your solar phase the wrong way. Sleeping into the morning hours will result in a sluggish Inner Climate®.

The Prep

If you have successfully exercised and regulated your caffeine consumption, very little prep is needed for this one. My only additional recommendation would be to avoid resting too much or napping during the day.

THE PRACTICE

Let every hour after 7pm slow you down. Start disengaging from the noise in the world and in your mind.

Go to bed by 9.45pm to turn out the lights by 10pm. You want to stick to this schedule for at least six out of seven days a week.

The Dilemmas

Attending social events

You may be part of a social circle that likes to meet late in the evenings. Would going to bed early mean losing your friends? As we start aging, most people increasingly begin to feel the negative side effects of going to sleep late, both in their bodies and moods. But just like you, they could possibly be stuck in the rut of needing to conform rather than being inspired to challenge the system. The truth is that we need disruptors if we want to save the planet and our own health.

At some point in my early thirties, I decided that late nights weren't working for me, especially on the weekdays. I would wake up dysfunctional and cranky and dampen the entire ecosystem with my moods. So, I became the disruptor among my friends. Instead of hanging out at a bar, I suggested we get tea, go for a foot massage, or meet earlier for a nature walk with our little ones in strollers. I was surprised by the reactions I received. More than willingness, there was relief. It seemed like everyone was waiting for someone else to say it. There were some who complained, who wanted to numb out their nights. I realized that leading a conscious life where I focused more on the long term, rather than fleeting short-term pleasures, would mean phasing out some of those friendships anyway, or at least meeting those friends on the weekends when I was more willing to play the late-night game.

Working the night shift
If your job keeps you up late, I feel for you. My first reaction would be to ask you to look for a daytime work opportunity, but you've probably already done that. Upon returning home from your night shift, whatever time it is, avoid the urge to eat a large meal or to spend time staring at a blue-lit screen. Instead, wash your face with water, drink a cup of hot milk or soup, massage your feet, and get into bed to minimize the damage. It's OK for you to sleep in, but you want to wake up to a solid, consistent morning routine, whenever that is. Oil massages are your best friend. Keep in mind that if you cannot follow the exogenous clock of the sun and moon, the next best thing would be to create a regular and consistent system of your own to reduce the load on your body.

Bed at 10pm is too early
If you're used to going to sleep after midnight, going to bed at 10pm could feel too early. But with a little bit of practice, regulation of caffeine, early dinners, regular exercise and a strong intention, it'll only be a matter of time before you get there. Ensure your room is slightly cool and dark, and that your bedding is heavy and cozy.

The night is my only private time

This can be true for many mothers with younger children. My first piece of advice is to move your kids to an earlier bedtime by 30 minutes. But, additionally, the night only feels precious because you haven't witnessed the peace, joy, and space that come with waking early. Try finding that extra hour in the mornings instead of at night. You'll learn that waking up early drastically enhances your efficiency for the entire day, while sleeping late can lower your productivity.

Change the narrative:
Instead of:
 "I couldn't wake up early because I slept late"
say:
 "I couldn't sleep late because I woke up early."

How many late nights is too many?

I understand that life happens, and we may have periods of many consecutive late nights. In my experience, the immune system gets affected after three back-to-back late nights, so resume going to sleep early after two late nights. It is also useful to get a massage when your sleep is compromised. If you are beginning to feel the dryness and soreness of going to bed late, try sleeping with a clove in your cheek's pocket. You read that right: sleeping with a clove (the spice) in your cheek's pocket. The clove will soften after a few minutes, and you won't be able to feel it, nor will you choke on it if you safely place it in the depths of your cheek. The oils from the clove will soothe your insides and help you wake up as good as new. This remedy also works wonders at the onset of a sore throat.

DAY 11
REGULATE YOUR WATER CONSUMPTION

The Wisdom

Consuming large amounts of water, especially when guzzled down quickly, significantly affects absorption and even dilutes the gastric juices. Water is received by the body's cells through absorption and osmosis, and hydration is more than just drinking water. Let me break it down for you.

Water traverses through your system and gets absorbed primarily in the small intestine through its semi-permeable membrane using the process of osmosis. This means that water moves to the other side of the small intestine and progresses through the different membranes into the cells, making its way from an area of low solute/salt concentration (the small intestine) to high solute/salt concentration (the cells). When a large amount of water is consumed, there is additional pressure on the body to absorb it quickly; this is an inefficient way to hydrate and distracts the body from other essential functions. Moreover, the kidneys must work harder to eliminate excess water from the system. At the same time, it can lead to dilution of sodium in the body and cause a condition called water intoxication, or hyponatremia, which can manifest as headache, nausea, fatigue, confusion, and muscle cramping. In certain cases, when not reversed quickly, it can lead to more life-threatening conditions. If you've ever watered a plant, you probably know that too much water can lead to waterlogging, mold, and poor water absorption.

At the same time, water has to pass through the stomach before it reaches the small intestine to be absorbed. Excess water dilutes the rich, warm environment of the stomach and disturbs the Inner Climate®. No wonder Ayurveda links drinking excess water to obesity. So, in that case, how should one hydrate?

You may recall from the "Bring in Moist" section on page 68 in Part 2 that the Ayurvedic recommendation for food intake is one-third solid, one-third liquid and the remaining third to be left vacant for the movement and churning of the food. The liquid and solid in equal proportions indicate that foods should be in a semi-solid state as far as possible. When foods with the appropriate amount of salt are consumed in a semi-solid state, the fluid portion gets absorbed in a manner that regulates the sodium to water proportions of the body. A soup is a great example of food that nourishes and hydrates simultaneously.

Herbal teas are also a great way to ensure that your body is not mechanically pushing water from membrane to membrane in the name of hydration. Firstly, the warm temperature of tea makes it difficult to drink fast, thereby preventing the dilution of gastric juices and regulating the pressure on the kidneys. At the same time, a warm beverage will dilate the blood vessels and channels and make absorption a bit easier in the body. Lastly, you can make tea with any herb that may serve an additional function in the body. For example, chamomile flowers soothe the digestive system and calm the nervous system, giving you more than just hydration.

This doesn't mean that you should never drink plain water, but plain water can be imbibed according to your levels of thirst. Healthy thirst can be quenched with just a few sips of water. Feeling excessively thirsty is normal if you're sweating profusely or in a very hot climate; in any other circumstance, excess thirst usually represents an imbalance in the system.

The Prep

If you've been switching out your cold beverage for warm tea since Day 5, you don't have much to prep for, but if you want to take it to the next level, think about what other herbs or herbal teas you want to experiment with. I recommend using loose organic herbs over anything in a tea sachet whenever possible.

THE PRACTICE

Continue the practice from Day 5.

1. Fill a 16 fl oz. (approx. 500ml) flask with hot water and herbs, cool it down to a temperature you can tolerate, pour it into a cup and sip it occasionally during the first half of the day. Note that sipping is different from drinking.

2. If you're done with the first flask before 4pm, fill another flask and drink what you can until 4pm. After 4pm, drink plain room-temperature water according to how thirsty you are, taking a few sips when needed. You can end your day with another cup of herbal tea if you wish.

3. As you try different herbs, notice the color, frequency, and quantity of your urine. Notice any other changes you experience.

The Dilemmas

Can I drink caffeinated tea for hydration?
Caffeinated tea is hot and dry, dehydrating the body. It is also a known diuretic, releasing water and salt through the urine, and it's not a replacement for herbal tea or water.

Drinking water with meals
Current research has shown that drinking water before meals can help weight loss in the short term by creating increased satiety.[6] Ayurvedic science agrees, but adds that consuming water right before a meal can deplete the body and may lead to unhealthy weight loss in the short term. Water before eating can dampen down the Agni and dilute its supporters, lowering appetite and, thus, the quantity of food needed, but creating inefficiencies in digestion and absorption. So, drinking water before meals is a no-go.

Drinking right after eating is also contraindicated. When we eat, blood rushes to the gut, activating the Agni and its supporters, and making things pretty fiery down there. But drinking water right after meals douses this fire and alters the Agni-enhanced climate of the gut that had geared up to break down your food. The dampened Agni slows down the process of food breakdown and leads to unhealthy weight gain, according to Ayurveda. However, drinking a few sips of hot water or herbal tea with your food can make chewing easier and even increase the blood flow to the gut, making digestion easier, and is a regular practice in several traditional Asian cultures.

Summer drinks
Staying hydrated during the summer takes on a whole new importance as the heat and humidity make us sweat more. This natural cooling mechanism helps regulate our body temperature and leads to the loss of vital water and electrolytes that must be replenished. But that's not all – sweating can

also dampen your appetite, creating a trifecta of challenges: dehydration, electrolyte imbalance, and decreased hunger.

Thankfully, we have two powerful allies: sour-tasting beverages and refreshing coconut water. The tangy flavor of sour drinks not only stimulates our digestive enzymes but triggers an immediate salivary response, revving up our metabolism, and quenching our thirst. Meanwhile, coconut water, nature's perfect antidote to a scorching day, comes packed with essential electrolytes, hydration, and nutrients, especially if you indulge in the delicious coconut meat nestled inside its protective shell.

Burning during urination

All my childhood summers were spent in the hot deserts of Rajasthan, India, where my maternal grandparents lived. Inevitably, by day three, I would start to experience intense burning during urination, and my mother would offer her antidote: to double down on beverages that contained rose water and rose jam. Soon enough, my hot and dry body would cool down and the rest of my summer would seem like a bed of roses, literally. It's not uncommon for those who live in extremely hot climates, or even those who possess a hot and dry Inner Climate®, to have a similar experience. You may need to play with the quantity of your water intake, adding cooling substances like rose water and rose buds, and stay open to some trial and error before you get it right.

Warm tea feels uncomfortable

There are those who instantly feel uncomfortable with drinking hot or warm water. If you can relate to this, you most likely experience symptoms in the upper digestive tract. You may have even played with explosive apple cider vinegar in the name of health. It may be a while before your body can build up its mucosal lining until it is comfortable with warm beverages. Feel free to cool your tea to room temperature and add mint to it for added soothing and cooling.

DAY 12
FATS WITHOUT FEAR

The Wisdom

Over the last several decades, more or less anything associated with the word "fat" has been stigmatized, whether it's fat in your food or fat on the body. While excess fat in both these places can cause the Inner Climate® to become stagnant and dense, appropriate amounts of fat are essential for the body to keep its lunar aspects intact. Fats are responsible for several building, protective, and repair functions. For example, fats are an important energy resource, providing more than twice the amount of energy per metric gram than proteins and carbohydrates do. Also, certain essential vitamins like A, D, E, and K are fat-soluble and can't be absorbed without the right intake of fats. Moreover, fats are key components of the cell membrane, maintaining the integrity and functionality of cells.

Our body constantly generates new cells and requires raw materials, including fats. Fats are also essential for our nervous system and brain health; our brain primarily comprises fats. Synthesis of hormones, especially those related to metabolism, reproduction, and stress, requires fats. Additionally, fats play a massive role in lubrication and insulation, helping to keep the body temperature within the desired range.

Our problematic relationship with fats was epitomized for me by Claire. Claire was 32 when she came to me for her panic attacks and the several phobias that she had developed over the last few years. As a young girl, she had felt some anxiety, but this hadn't prevented her from functioning well at school. Growing up, she had a moderate frame and never thought much about it till she moved to the US from Hungary in her early twenties.

In the US, she was amazed to find low-fat versions of everything and quickly bought into it all. While she didn't feel great in her gut with this new change, she was willing to pay the price for a lower dress size. But it didn't stop there; she moved on to a high-protein diet and water fasting. In the last four months, she had consumed no more than one small bottle of olive oil.

Beneath her makeup, her face looked gaunt and her skin patchy. I noticed facial and vocal tics as she spoke, something she had developed in the last five years. Lack of fats and imbalanced nourishment had created havoc with her Inner Climate®, leaving it parched, windy, and depleted. Her gut was lifeless and her nervous system was about to short-circuit. But before therapy, she needed fats. Initially, rather than adding them back into her diet, I asked her to introduce daily oil massage into her life. Eventually, we moved on to belly-button oiling (see page 202), and hair oiling (see page 219). When she became friends with oil, we increased the amount of fats she used in her existing foods; we threw out all the low-fat versions. She began to sleep and feel better. In conjunction with therapy and herbs, she eventually restored some sense of equilibrium.

While Claire's story is extreme, I see elements of her reality in many of the stories I hear daily. Fats are like friends: If you choose the right ones, they make your life significantly better, whereas the wrong type are destructive.

Before I discuss useful fats, I'm going to talk about harmful fats. Highly processed fats like hydrogenated trans-fats (found in fried foods, baked goods, processed foods, and margarine, for example) get dumped into the bloodstream, increasing LDL cholesterol and decreasing HDL cholesterol. LDL, commonly referred to as bad cholesterol, can increase buildup of plaque that can block arteries. HDL, on the other hand, is referred to as good cholesterol and generally does the opposite by removing plaque from the arteries to the liver to be metabolized. Saturated fats found in fatty meat, butter, and cheese can also increase LDL.

Low-fat versions of common food items can also be highly processed. Not only that, but foods that are usually labeled as low fats can often be very dry and dense, lacking moisture and leading to clogging and constipation. I personally have never bought a snack or food item that read zero-fat or low-fat on the label. I stick to warm and moist as much as possible.

In contrast, monounsaturated fats found in avocados, olive oil, almonds, and other nuts can lower LDL and support HDL. Polyunsaturated fats found in fatty fish, walnuts, flaxseed, and sunflower oil, for example, are also essential for brain function and cell growth.

Ghee is an exception and doesn't act like most fats in spite of being a saturated fat. The primary reason for this is that ghee is made from cultured butter. The culturing process provides the warm and moist qualities of fermentation and supports ghee's breakdown of the fats. Ghee can, in fact, support digestion and heart health. It also carries all the essential nutritional value of milk, yet without the casein and the lactose, the two hardest components of milk to break down. (You will find other benefits of ghee described in Part 2, page 70.)

The Prep

Buy a bottle of good-quality extra virgin olive oil and a jar of organic cultured ghee. Throw out any snacks or foods labeled "low-fat" or "zero-fat." Instead, buy some high-quality organic almonds, walnuts, pumpkin seeds, and sunflower seeds.

THE PRACTICE

Include fats in all your three main meals: breakfast, lunch, and dinner.

Start cooking by warming a good fat on low heat and tempering it with appropriate spices. Traditionally, all Ayurvedic recipes start with blooming cumin and turmeric in warm ghee before the main ingredients are added. (We will talk more about blooming spices on Day 13.)

Sprinkle pumpkin and sunflower seeds on any vegetables and foods that you think they would pair well with. Drizzle olive oil on vegetables or on toasted sourdough. Basically, become fearless with the right fats.

The Dilemmas

I'm not used to ghee

If ghee is not something you are used to, go slow. Start by using 1 teaspoon in a single meal, then increase this to using it in two or more meals daily over a few weeks. Over time, you can increase the quantity of ghee per meal. Notice if you feel heavy or sluggish after consuming ghee or see slime in your stools; that may be a sign that you have gone too far and need to cut down the quantity. It's important to monitor changes in your cholesterol as you introduce new fats into your diet. Blooming some turmeric powder (a few pinches per teaspoon) in warm ghee and curry leaves (1 chopped curry leaf per teaspoon) in the ghee can make it easier for it to be broken down to benefit the body.

Sluggish Inner Climate®

If you have identified your Inner Climate® as sluggish and your body has excess adipose tissue, you want to watch your fat intake. Cut out all processed fats and reserve fat for cooking with olive oil and ghee. You can include a small amount of soaked nuts and some seeds in your diet. It is important for you to add spices to your fats while cooking. Exercising will also help you to put your fats to the right use.

Cooking fat

The world of cooking fats has become a difficult place to navigate. Oils that were once deemed safe to use are now being processed in a way that makes them harmful. I would recommend four cooking fats, with the first two being my go-tos.

1. **Ghee:** Ghee has a high smoke point and can be used for sautéing, frying, and even baking, as long as your body is used to it.

2. **Extra virgin olive oil:** Great when you need to stir-fry and sauté at low to moderate heats.

3. **Extra virgin sesame oil:** This can be heated to quite a high heat. While it can be used occasionally throughout the year and a little more frequently in the winter months, use sparingly if your Inner Climate® is on the hotter side.

4. **Coconut oil:** If you are used to cooking in coconut oil, you can continue to do so, especially in the summer months. Coconut oil is a good choice when you want to change it up or if you are vegan but your Inner Climate® is hot and you want to use it instead of ghee.

DAY 13
SPICE IT UP

The Wisdom

Ayurveda believes spices can help speed up the metabolism not just in your body but in your food. Spices support the breakdown of food even before you consume them, making them a key ingredient in every Ayurvedic recipe. Also, most spices contain micro-nutrients and are antioxidant and anti-inflammatory, and several are antimicrobial and can even regulate blood sugar levels and cholesterol. No wonder Ayurvedic food can be treated as medicine!

Essential substances that the modern world of nutrition systematically consumes in the form of supplements are built naturally into the Ayurvedic diet through the use of spices, so you can enjoy their health benefits and savor their flavor at the same time. In fact, those traditional cultures around the world that have understood a thing or two about health also have a long track record of using spices in their food. Spices keep the Inner Climate® warm, the Agni fired up and foods on track to be broken down. However, not all spices are equal, and I strongly recommend not using them on their own. Spices are potent, hot, and dry, and, as we saw in Part 2, can easily burn your Inner Climate® unless diluted by fats or food. There are four ways to use them effectively:

1. **Boil:** To support their breakdown, add whole spices to grains, legumes, and other foods during the cooking process. I love to throw in a bay leaf, a short cinnamon stick, a clove, or a cardamom pod while boiling rice, lentils, or other starchy foods such as potatoes. My choice of spice depends on the flavors I am going for.

2. **Bloom:** Whole spices like cumin, mustard seeds, caraway, carom, and others can be bloomed in a good fat at the start of the cooking process. This involves warming a good fat over a medium flame, adding approximately ⅛th of a teaspoon per spice per serving, and allowing these to simmer in the fat for a few seconds, while being careful not to burn them. Other items that require cooking can then be added to this fat–spice base. You can change the spices' quantities depending on your needs. Some ground spices like asafetida and turmeric can also be bloomed. Blooming activates the spices and can even improve their efficacy.

3. **Flavor/ sprinkle:** Some ground spices can be added even later in the cooking process. Roasted cumin, turmeric, ginger powder, coriander seed powder, and paprika, for example, are often added later in the cooking process. Similarly, oregano, thyme, black pepper, and cinnamon can be used as table spices with which to sprinkle food after cooking.

4. **Tea:** Spices can also be consumed in a steeped tea or boiled in hot water. Boiling increases their potency, so be careful not to overheat your system. Depending on my goal, I often choose between using fennel seeds, carom seeds, or ginger powder in my tea.

Remember that a good spice shouldn't burn on your tongue. Besides dilution, there are a few rules when using spices, so play with them and see how your palate and gut respond to them.

The Prep

Spend 45 to 60 minutes familiarizing yourself with spices in a food market or a health food store. Smell them and get a sense of their flavor; what foods or cuisines would you want to try them in? Read their labels and learn about their origins and traditional use. Meet them in-person first, even if you eventually end up buying your spices online.

Below is a list of 10 essential spices with their benefits and uses.

Key to table
- **Benefits:** While most spices have innumerable benefits, the Benefits column in the table below lists the most relevant ones. All spices will boost Agni and support the digestion of food, and most can be anti-inflammatory and antimicrobial when consumed correctly; hence, these two benefits are assumed and not listed below.
- **Warmth level:** Some spices are inherently more warming than others. The ones marked with three stars are the warmest, so use them judiciously in smaller quantities. Keep an eye out for acne or any other heat-led symptoms.
- **Uses:** This column explains how to use these spices easily and effectively. However, feel free to experiment a little.
- **Recommended cuisine or foods:** Experimenting with spices can feel quite daunting, especially if you aren't really a Julia Child. This column tells you the cuisines that the spice is commonly paired with. Once again, feel free to play with these suggestions.

I suggest purchasing small jars or quantities of each spice in the first instance. Remember that cooking is intuitive, so trust your instincts and set an intention to befriend every ingredient.

ESSENTIAL SPICE LIST				
Spice	Benefits	Warmth Level	Uses	Recommended Cuisine or Foods
Ginger	Detox, food and nutrient assimilation	**	Tea, flavor, sprinkle	All
Cinnamon powder	Blood sugar regulation, weight management, antioxidant	*	Flavor, sprinkle	Non-savory foods, desserts, Middle Eastern and Indian cuisines
Carom seeds	Exceptional for bloating, metabolism, appetite stimulant, colds, detoxes, useful in menstrual cramps	***	Bloom Bloating and menstrual cramps: consume ½tsp with 7 to 8 pinches of Himalayan pink salt and drink with warm water	Indian, Middle Eastern, Mexican, marinara sauce, cruciferous vegetables
Cumin seeds	Anti-flatulent, weight loss, disintegrates and digests mucus, menstrual cramps	**	Bloom, flavor	Indian, Middle Eastern, Mexican, Ethiopian
Bay leaf	Antioxidant, antimicrobial, menstrual cramps, helpful in breaking down cholesterol	*	Boil, bloom	Indian, Mediterranean, French, Italian, Spanish, Middle Eastern, Eastern European

ESSENTIAL SPICE LIST				
Spice	**Benefits**	**Warmth Level**	**Uses**	**Recommended Cuisine or Foods**
Powdered turmeric	Lowers excesses (e.g. of cholesterol, diabetes), pain relief, invigorates blood circulation, powerful antioxidant	**	Flavor, bloom	Indian, Middle Eastern, South East Asian
Black pepper	Enhances bio-availability of other substances, antimicrobial, fat loss, unclogs respiratory channels	**	Flavor, sprinkle	All
Cloves	Alleviates nausea, pain relief, boosts immunity, fungal infections, heart health	**	Bloom, boil, flavor, sprinkle, tea	Indian, Middle Eastern, South East Asian, South American
Coriander seeds	Detox, relieves indigestion, regulates blood sugar, antimicrobial, antispasmodic	*	Bloom, tea	Indian, Middle Eastern, South East Asian, Latin
Cardamom Seeds	Relieves nausea, soothes throat, freshens breath, reduces oral bacteria, regulates cholesterol, mood and cognitive function	**	Boil, bloom, tea, flavor	Indian, Middle Eastern, Thai, Persian, Scandinavian, Turkish

Below is a Level 2 spice list of ingredients that you can experiment with if you want to spice things up even further. While you don't need to graduate to this next list, I want you to have it should you choose to explore further.

LEVEL 2 SPICE LIST				
Spice	Benefits	Warmth Level	Uses	Recommended Cuisine or Foods
Mustard Seeds	Expectorant, antimicrobial, circulation, unclogs channels	***	Bloom	Indian Subcontinent, South East Asian, Mediterranean, European, German, French
Asafetida	Constipation, reduces gas, antimicrobial and antifungal, antioxidant	***	Bloom, flavor (use no more than a small pinch)	Indian, Iranian
Saffron	Stimulates appetite, enhances mood and cognitive function	***	Soak in milk or water before use	A couple of strands soaked for a rich, aromatic flavor
Coriander seed powder	Similar to coriander seeds but more flavor	*	Flavor	Indian, Middle Eastern, Thai, Mexican, Latin
Pomegranate seed powder	Relieves acidity, soothes inflammation, can help in migraines, detoxes, antioxidant	Cooling	Flavor, boil, tea	Use for tartness in any cuisines, great with lentils, Middle Eastern, Indian, Mediterranean, Moroccan, Mexican

LEVEL 2 SPICE LIST				
Spice	Benefits	Warmth Level	Uses	Recommended Cuisine or Foods
Amla powder	Soothes hyperacidity, antioxidant, blood sugar regulation, eye health, immune support (vitamin C)	Cooling	Flavor, boil	Use for tart flavor

THE PRACTICE

1. Start to include spices in all your foods. If your breakfast is oatmeal, add a dash of cinnamon. If you eat sweet potatoes, throw in a cinnamon stick while boiling; use black pepper on your avocados. Throw in a clove or a bay leaf to everything that requires boiling.

2. You may take to some spices instantly and realize that some aren't for you yet, and that's fine. But you'll never know till you try.

The Dilemmas

Kitchen smells
While spices seem aromatic, they can leave a peculiar smell in your kitchen. So make sure to have an air vent or a window open. Deodorize your home occasionally by lighting some naturally scented nontoxic candles or incense sticks.

Quantities

Start small and tune in to the flavors of spices and their potential impact on your body before you go all out. Ideally, start with one small piece of a whole spice like cloves or cinnamon and only a few pinches of powdered spices before moving up to the ⅛th teaspoon per serving.

Strong taste

If you cannot get used to the taste of a certain spice, let it go. Choose another one. Spices are so versatile and three are so many options, you can probably get the same benefits from a spice that suits your palate better.

ADJUST YOUR SHOWER TEMPERATURE

The Wisdom

When my youngest started preschool in 2015, I suddenly had two precious hours of downtime. There were many things I could have done with that time, but I chose to hurry back home every day after drop-off to take a long shower. If you're the mother of young children, you can probably relate to that luxury. Right there, in my small shower, I found heaven every single day.

As the weather got colder, my water temperature got hotter and my showers became longer. I remember walking out of the shower one day, surprised to see the redness on my skin; it looked like the start of a sunburn and settled down soon enough. By the time I was on the other side of autumn, my skin had lost all its moisture and became extremely parched and lifeless. That winter wasn't exceptionally cold for others, but for me, it was hard on my body. It was almost like my body had forgotten how to thermoregulate, and my extremities were always cold and my skin was always itchy.

The Ayurvedically aware part of me knew where this imbalance was coming from, but I told myself every day that this would be the last day of my hot showers. What finally motivated me to shift gears was when my luscious hair became lifeless, like straw.

According to Ayurveda, showers or baths are meant to be taken with lukewarm to warm water. They may not be as relaxing as hot-water showers, but they gently open the pores and cleanse the body while maintaining the integrity of the skin barrier. However, an even milder water temperature is recommended for the chest area and above, in order to protect the heart region from overheating.

The Prep

Exercise before you shower so that you are warmed up, but wait for your breathing to return to normal and for your body to regain its equilibrium before you jump into the shower.

THE PRACTICE

Take showers or baths with warm water rather than hot water. For the chest and head region, you may go even milder.

This practice can take a few days to adapt to, but once you do, you'll notice the huge difference it makes to your blood circulation, thermoregulation, skin, and hair.

The Dilemmas

Hot tubs

I may not care much for swimming pools when I travel, but a hot tub is always at the top of my list of indulgences. However, it's only an indulgence, not something I do every day. If you're like me, feel free to soak in a hot tub occasionally, but for no more than 10 to 15 minutes at a time.

That being said, the sulfuric therapeutic spring baths were the original hot tubs. Although warmer than the recommended temperature, they offer therapeutic benefits due to the presence of sulfur and magnesium and can be used a little more leniently if you have access to one. Even then, the chest and head region are always kept above water to prevent overheating.

Skin conditions

If you have a skin condition that is accompanied by an itch or rash, you need to be even more mindful of your hot water usage. Hot water often aggravates hives or allergic reactions. Sulfuric water may be useful for you, but I recommend working with a practitioner to determine what treatments are suitable.

DAY 15
ABHYANGA SELF-LOVE

The Wisdom

Abhyanga involves massaging your body with oil, and is the ultimate practice of self-love. In the Ayurvedic world, the skin is viewed as a channel of consumption and oil is its food. Many skin microbes are lipophilic, which means they can break down fat and create byproducts that have antimicrobial properties or moisturize the skin. So, oiling is your defense against pathogens, strengthening your inner army. Abhyanga should ideally be performed before you shower, as this will also protect you from the damage that water can potentially cause to the skin barrier.

Abhyanga promotes self-touch and helps the body release oxytocin, the love hormone. Thus, it helps to regulate and comfort the nervous system. Ayurveda believes that abhyanga is also an anti-aging practice that strengthens the body, slows down wear and tear, and repairs damage caused by UV rays and free radicals.

Ayurvedic texts are loaded with paragraphs on the benefits of abhyanga that go beyond the ones stated above, including restful sleep, reduction of anxiety, better blood circulation, and even nourishment of deeper tissues.

Ideally, abhyanga should be performed with warm oil before exercise so that oil can penetrate the body's channels and nourish its deep tissues when the body warms up during the workout. Moreover, since the skin is a channel of consumption, this is your food before you exercise. You'll be surprised how well the oil can sustain you when absorbed in this way, without the need to consume any through your mouth.

The Prep

Buy yourself a good-quality body oil, ideally without any strong or artificial fragrance. Ayurveda recommends sesame oil, but coconut oil may be better suited if your body has inflammation or if you live in a very hot climate. If you can get your hands on Ayurvedic massage oils, even better. If you choose to go all the way, buy yourself a bottle warmer to warm up the oil before you let your body soak in its goodness.

THE PRACTICE

Warm the oil in a bottle warmer by simply throwing the bottle in for a few minutes. Take some oil and massage your entire body, starting with the belly button and then around your abdomen in a clockwise direction, moving on to your shoulders and limbs, with massage strokes in the direction of the body hair.

Make sure to cover every inch of your body, ideally maintaining contact with your skin throughout. At this stage, the technique is not so important; get comfortable with the feeling of oil on your body and let your practice find its way, day by day.

If you have the space for it, keep a little stool in your bathroom to sit on to make your practice more comfortable and easy.

As mentioned, abhyanga should ideally be performed before exercise and/or showering. Before you exercise, wipe down your palms and the soles of your feet so you don't slip.

Abhyanga can last for as few as 5 minutes or a more extended 45-minute practice; I assure you that it's one practice that you won't want to give up once you start.

The Dilemmas

Abhyanga contraindications

Avoid abhyanga altogether if you have a skin condition like a rash, eczema, or psoriasis. If you live in a very hot and humid climate or are in the middle of a hot summer, skip this practice. If you are sick with a fever, indigestion, or even a cold, wait until you fully recover as you may not have the metabolic ability to process the oil. If you are on your period or pregnant, this may not be the best time to perform abhyanga.

Exercising with oil

Getting used to exercising when covered in oil can take some practice, and sweating may make it even more uncomfortable. There are a couple things that may help. First, try using less oil and massaging deeper so your skin can absorb the oil before you exercise. If not, try wiping down any excesses with a towel reserved for this purpose. If that still doesn't work, oil your joints before exercise and then massage the rest of your body right before you shower.

I don't have the time to perform a full abhyanga

I believe in creating shorter versions of every ritual in case you find yourself in a day when 24 hours seem too few. To shorten your abhyanga practice, skip the full-body massage and oil your joints, belly button, the crown of the head, behind the ears, and the soles of your feet before you jump into the shower.

Abhyanga after shower

We are used to moisturizing after showering, so why can't we use abhyanga then instead? Firstly, being naked in the shower increases our need for moisturizing since water can affect the skin barrier by stripping the essential oils and leaving us drier afterwards. But when you take your oiled body into the shower, the oil protects the skin barrier from that damage. At the same time, it reduces the need for moisturizing afterward. That being said, if you were to oil your body after you come out of the shower or bath, there's a high chance that it could clog your pores and even make you prone to infection. However, if you have very dry skin and find a lighter, less dense oil, make an exception and use it occasionally after your shower.

DAY 16
NASYA YOUR NOSE

The Wisdom

Inserting oil drops into one's nose isn't a commonplace practice in modern times, but it's Ayurveda's secret sauce for brain health and beyond. Food and exercise usually nourish the bulk of our body, including the neck and below. But our head, neck, and sensory organs are often neglected. However, our nose and the rest of the respiratory region are just as important for good health as our digestion system, if not more so.

We take in food through the mouth and oxygen through our breath, both critical for life. But if your nasal passages are clogged and slimy, the microbiome in there is affected and you can find yourself repeatedly getting sick and even compromise how effectively your body receives oxygen. Nasya drops can create a warm and moist environment for the microbiome to thrive, making you less prone to airborne disease. It also helps in rhinitis, tonsillitis, and other conditions of the ENT region.

Not only this, but nasya's benefits extend to the deepest corners of this area. The nasal passages bypass the blood–brain barrier and reach parts of the brain that cannot be accessed otherwise. Medical research is currently being conducted to explore the nasal route for drug administration to the brain, especially for conditions such as Alzheimer's and

Parkinson's.[7,8] The practice of nasya supports brain health and function, and Ayurvedic doctors believe that it may even prevent the onset of certain neurological disorders. Moreover, nasya is also useful for treating throat pain, headaches, and jaw, neck, and shoulder stiffness.

Prep

You can buy a bottle of Anu Taila, a herbal nasal drop used for nasya, from an Ayurvedic store or from a reputable vendor online.

PRACTICE

Warm the whole nasya bottle by placing it in a bowl of hot water.

Once the bottle is slightly warm to the touch, lie down flat with your head slightly tilted back and a pillow placed underneath your neck.

Insert just two drops of warm nasya oil in each nostril. Do not snort; let the oil gradually make its way down into your nasal passage.

Wait a couple of minutes before you get up and get going again.

You may feel the need to expectorate. It's a good thing; the nasya decongests sticky, stubborn phlegm. Let it out.

Avoid jumping into the shower for the next 30 minutes.

Dilemmas

Nasya tastes funny
Nasya oil can, and probably should, drip down into your throat, and it can take a while to get used to this. But it's also indicative of just how far a couple of drops can travel. In the same way that they make it to your throat, they're also traveling in the other direction to your brain, so hurray!

Nasya feels itchy and burns
Nasya oil can burn, especially if the mucosal lining in your nose is compromised. It usually takes a week or two for the nasal environment to start changing and for the oil to feel milder. That being said, if the nasya feels itchy or burns in your throat, gargle with warm water, making sure that the gargling water reaches all the way to your throat. You can also wash your face with cool water for relief.

I'm always congested
If you're always congested, nasya may be your savior. However, you may want to start by inhaling some steam from an ionic facial steamer. I usually like to keep one on my bathroom counter so that I can inhale steam while brushing my teeth.

Once the phlegm has loosened, massage the sinuses around your nose in a circular motion, moving outward to the side of the temples. Repeat this with the sinuses above the eyebrows. Make this intuitive; remember, your body already knows. You will feel the area that needs to be massaged in order to loosen the phlegm and get it moving further.

If you're used to practicing neti (a type of nasal cleanse), this is the time to do it. Wait 20 to 30 minutes afterwards before you put your nasya drops in. This protocol has worked wonders for several of my clients who have been chronically congested. The one disclaimer is that neti salt can be corrosive to the insides, so practice neti on no more than three days a week.

I can't obtain Anu Taila oil

If Anu Taila is unavailable, you can start by using plain sesame oil for nasya, as mentioned earlier.

DAY 17
BEFRIEND YOUR BREATH

The Wisdom

From my earliest memories, my breath has been my closest companion, even before I made real friends. My mother's remedy for all of life's challenges was simple: "Bring awareness to your breath." Whether it concerned my fear of the dark, frustration with math problems, a tummy ache, or even the whims of a child's imagination, her advice was always the same. Through her, I discovered a world of healing and emotional processing long before I understood those concepts.

And remember how, on the 10-day silent Vipassana meditation retreat that I went on when I was a teenager, we spent 13 hours each day simply becoming present with our breath? By the third day, my awareness had sharpened to the point where I could detect which nostril was active, even in my sleep. This experience was transformative and ignited a lifelong exploration of the breath.

Over the years, I have explored various practices, from holotropic breathwork to becoming a certified pranayama instructor. Pranayama is a branch of yoga that focuses on manipulating the breath to enhance prana, or life force. This mastery allowed me to deliver both my babies in a state of complete calm, without uttering a single shriek, as I used my breath to disconnect from my body yet stay anchored in my consciousness.

I will be encouraging you to embark on your own journey with the breath and let it take you to places that you could have never imagined, but first let's revisit some key insights that were briefly mentioned in the chapter "Your Toolkit," on page 127.

The nose is for breathing and the mouth is for eating, so the ideal is to breathe through the nose. Our nostrils act like filters, preventing dust, allergens, and microbes from making it into our respiratory system. Moreover, nasal breathing warms and moistens the air before it reaches the lungs, thereby improving lung function and our overall respiratory health. Ooh! How warm and moist! Our nasal passages also produce nitric oxide, which has antimicrobial properties and helps to enhance oxygen uptake in the lungs. Nasal breathing also promotes better use of the diaphragm, leading to deeper, more efficient breaths and supporting better oxygen exchange and circulation throughout the body.

In addition to this, our breath tells us about our current state of mind. When we feel triggered or panic, the breath becomes short and rapid. Just becoming present with it changes its course and, as a result, resets the nervous system. When we are rested and relaxed, the breath deepens. And if you were to fall into a subconscious state, the breath would become very subtle, almost absent. You can use your breath to detect the onset of an emotional trigger and use awareness to bring it back into a state of calm without getting sucked into the trigger vortex.

I personally avoid making major decisions when my breathing is short and rapid. Decisions from that intense place feel strong and intuitive, but are impulsive since the nervous system is not in equilibrium. I wait for the breath to regulate and to return as a whole to a warm and moist state. I have found that decisions made in this manner feel clear, organic, and intuitive.

This is also a good time to pick up our earlier conversation and explore the shifts the body experiences with each inhale and exhale. Each inhale puts the body in sympathetic state. For our purposes, let's call this the solar or "doing" mode. In contrast, each exhalation puts the body in the parasympathetic, lunar or "being" mode. Ideally, as we saw in Part 1, we want to balance our doing with being and our solar with lunar. However, when we are constantly in a doing mode, we shorten our exhalations, and as a result, our breath dysregulates. When the body has had enough, it forces out a sigh, which is nothing but a long exhale. But by bringing awareness to our breath and actively expanding the exhales while we are busy, we can keep the mind in a state of flow – in a state of "being" while we are also "doing." Pretty incredible!

You may also recall from an earlier section that our left and right nostrils also have unique energies. Even though our bodies may look perfectly symmetrical externally, the world inside us is quite divided. The right and left brains have unique abilities; the right-side organs (such as the liver, gallbladder, and appendix) have more metabolic abilities than the left (e.g. the heart and spleen). Similarly, the right nostril carries solar energies, and the left nostril carries lunar energies. When they are balanced, the body is in the perfect place, warm and moist.

Balancing our inhalations and exhalations tends to restore warmth and moisture in the mind, while the balance of the right and left nostrils has a little more to do with the state of the body and the circadian rhythm. For example, it is natural for most people to have a more active right nostril during the peak of the day.

Shefali, my 17-year-old niece, has always been a bright girl. She is the sharpest in the room, but it's obvious that her body is hot and dry. With her dry and hot eczema patches, charred winter lips, high-pitched and piercing voice, and bouts of constipation since childhood, she could be a hot and dry case study. Growing up, she also constantly complained of a blocked nostril. Upon asking, I discovered that her left (lunar) nostril was perpetually blocked due to a deviated nasal septum. It all added up: Her chronically active right nostril had solarized her body.

The Prep

Download the free Breathing App created by Eddie Stern at www.thebreathing.app and get ready to play with your breath.

THE PRACTICE

Actively bring your awareness to the natural flow of your breath several times a day. If you can catch yourself at the start of a trigger vortex and notice the shifts in your breath, continue to observe it till it feels settled.

In addition to this, pick at least one of the two following practices to add to your morning routine. If you can do both, even better:

1. *Resonance breath:* Using the Breathing App, set an inhale–exhale ratio, and follow along with the gong for four minutes. Make sure that you're breathing through your nose. This breathing practice balances the inhalations and exhalations, expands your breath, relaxes your being, and increases prana. Sometimes, I like to use the app even while I am working. My subconscious mind takes cues from the gong and enhances my exhales, allowing me to think more clearly and be more efficient without burning out.

2. *Alternate nostril breathing:* This is a restorative practice, and you can feel the immediate benefits of the calm it brings. While the original practice requires the fingers to be in a specific position or *mudra*, I will simplify this and break it down so you can at least get started. As you read this, try to practice it at the same time to familiarize yourself with the practice.

3. Block your right nostril with your right thumb and breathe in through the left nostril slowly, counting to 6.

4. Close both nostrils (right thumb blocking the right nostril and right middle and fourth fingers blocking the left nostril) and hold for a count of 12.

5. Let go of the right thumb and exhale from the right for a count of 12.

6. Now, with the left nostril blocked (still with your right middle and fourth fingers), breathe in through the right nostril for a count of 6.

7. Hold once again for 12 counts and exhale, this time from the left nostril for a count of 12.

8. This completes one cycle.

Read these instructions and practice the breath once more to internalize it.

Bring the practice to your morning routine; do four complete rounds with your eyes closed every day. You can repeat the practice again at night or anytime during the day you need a reset, as long as you aren't carrying the fresh weight of a meal in your tummy.

Dilemmas and Notes

Holotropic breathing

The idea of exploring one's breath is fairly new to the Western world, and people may confuse the benefits of one practice with another. Holotropic breathing is very different from the type of breathwork mentioned above. Holotropic breathing is specifically designed to take you into other realms of consciousness, even to work through trauma and release it, as well as to free up trapped energies. This sort of breathing practice is best done under the guidance of a breathwork expert.

Kapal bhati and other forms of pranayama

If you have explored other branches of yoga, you may have stumbled upon other forms of pranayama like *kapal bhati, brahmari,* or *bhastrika. Brahmari* is safe to practice independently and can even be added to your morning routine. If you want to explore anything beyond that, work with a pranayama expert to design a practice that suits you.

OIL SWISHING

The Wisdom

The practice of swishing oil in the mouth may sound odd, but you have to try it to understand the benefits fully. By now, you've probably guessed that Ayurvedic science believes in oiling everything you can. My mantra is "ghee in your body, oil on your body." Oil creates the perfect warm and moist environment for a healthy and happy microbiome. And by now, even modern science concurs that when the microbiome thrives, we thrive.

The mouth is rich in bacteria, and you want this to be of the friendly variety. The main benefits of oil swishing (also known as oil pulling) are replacing the microbiome and preventing tooth decay, gum inflammation, and bad breath. But beyond that, oil swishing can possibly strengthen your jaws, relax jaw tightness, reduce facial puffiness, prevent tooth and gum sensitivity, tone the cheek muscles, and help prevent dryness in the throat and the cracking of lips. My mother swears that her teeth have become whiter and stronger since she started oil swishing. You may think oil swishing sounds too good to be true, so I want you to try it yourself; don't just believe me. The changes will become noticeable after about three weeks of consistent practice.

The Prep

If you haven't already done so for the earlier practices, I'd like you to buy yourself a bottle of expeller-pressed, organic sesame oil. Also, buy a cooking oil dispenser with a spout. Pour your sesame oil into the dispenser and keep it ready on your bathroom counter.

THE PRACTICE

After brushing your teeth and tongue scraping, put about 1 tablespoon (15ml) of oil in your mouth, tilt your head gently upward, and swish from side to side for a few minutes, ideally until you feel the oiliness in your nose and eyes. Spit it out once you've done this.

Wash your face with cool water afterward and rinse your mouth with plain water. If you feel the urge to brush your teeth, go ahead and do it.

The Dilemmas

Oil swishing modified for the modern day

I acknowledge that adding a bundle of practices to your day in a short period can feel overwhelming, so let me share my modified oil swishing practice with you. Without tilting your head backward, try swishing a little oil around your mouth for about five to seven minutes. You can do this while you're in the shower or even putting on your clothes. Multitasking may make it easier to bring this practice into your life.

Clogging drains
Oil will clog your drains and even your toilet bowl, if that is where you decide to dispose of it. I've found that spitting out the oil into small disposable bags which I can then put in the trash is the easiest and most practical solution.

Mouth ulcers, soreness, or gingivitis
If you have mouth ulcers or any soreness, avoid oil swishing and use cool cow's milk instead. If you don't actively have ulcers but are prone to them, try coconut oil instead of sesame oil and see how that works out for you. Similarly, if you are prone to gingivitis, experiment with coconut oil.

DAY 19
HEAD ABHYANGA

The Wisdom

The head is home to the brain, several control centers of the body and mind, and the nervous system's headquarters. Even though the world has taken to head abhyanga for its hair benefits, hair abhyanga actually nourishes the head, quickly relaxes the nervous system, and promotes restful sleep. If you've ever had someone run their fingers through your hair or even give you a scalp massage, you'll know what I mean. Hair abhyanga is one of my favorite practices, and I do it religiously twice a week.

Head abhyanga also enhances the quality of your hair and promotes new hair growth. You see, our hair grows in follicles that channel natural oils called sebum. As we age and expose our hair to wind, sun, stress, heat, and styling products, the sebum starts to dry out and the grounding of the hair in the follicle loosens. This can result in dry and frizzy hair and hair loss. Hair oil replenishes the lost oils and is akin to food for the hair.

I also use hair oil as a pre-conditioner, as I need a protectant for my hair before I expose it to the hard water of NYC. This eliminates the need for me to condition it afterward.

The Prep
You can start with just the sesame oil you may have already bought for previous practices or buy a special Ayurvedic hair oil. The ingredients you want to look for in the oil are brahmi, indigo, alma, and bhringraj.

THE PRACTICE

Head abhyanga can be performed anywhere from 20 minutes to 2 hours before you wash your hair.

1.   Untangle your hair and part it neatly. Apply warm oil with a dropper or a cotton bud along the length of the parting. Massage it in with your fingertips.

2.   Continue to part your hair all along the sides of your head and apply the oil over all lengths where it's been parted.

3.   Once you feel that oil has covered every area of your scalp, put the bottle aside and massage your scalp, dragging your fingertips in a circular motion. Breathe deeply as you do this and massage intuitively for five to seven minutes.

4.   Apply some more oil generously to the ends of your hair and massage it in. Enjoy the sense of grounding and relaxation the practice brings you before you wash your hair.

5.   Wash it off and repeat the practice once a week.

Dilemmas and Notes

Washing off the hair oil

If washing off the hair oil requires a lot of shampoo, isn't it counterproductive? Yes, it is. Use only a small quantity of oil if you find you need to use extra shampoo to remove any excess oil. Personally, I use a gram flour rinse that instantly helps to get the oils out of the hair without the chemicals of a shampoo. To do this, take a tablespoon of gram flour (a flour made from chickpeas) in a big bowl to your shower. Add a few cups of water to the gram flour in the shower and mix using your fingers. Pour this rinse on the top of your head. The dry gram flour will instantly start absorbing the oil. Without waiting a second, rinse out the gram flour in the shower. Do not wait even for a few seconds, as it can become very dry. Use a sparing amount of shampoo to remove any remaining excess oil.

Sleeping with hair oil

If you are used to this practice, you might like to try keeping on the hair oil overnight. I personally love to sleep with the oil, as it promotes restful and deep sleep. Just remember to keep a special pillow cover reserved for this purpose, or cover your pillow with a towel.

Hair oil in winter

Avoid stepping out in the cold winter air with oil in your hair, especially if it has a coconut oil base. Coconut oil has thick lipids and can quickly solidify, leaving you uncomfortable and perhaps even leading to the onset of congestion. If you find that oiling always leads to congestion, buy an Ayurvedic oil without a coconut base. If that also doesn't work for you, you probably can't metabolize the oil. In that case, feel free to do a dry scalp massage.

Hair oiling as a bonding family tradition

Traditionally, hair oiling has been a family bonding tradition. Usually, the mothers and grandmothers of the household will perform a head abhyanga for the younger ones and each other. When I was growing up, my aunts and my mother oiled my hair, and right up to the present day, I have almost always managed to recruit someone to do my abhyanga. It's also my privilege to pass on this nourishing practice to my daughters and I'll carry on performing a head abhyanga for them as often as they are ready to receive it.

DAY 20
FOOT MASSAGE

The Wisdom

Traditional Chinese Medicine believes that the feet are a microcosm of the body, with each area corresponding to an organ system or bodily area. The feet are also the end point of several meridians – the subtle channels believed to carry qi or life force, akin to prana.

Ayurveda, too, believes that the feet carry significant marma points. Marma points are energy centers rich in the flow of prana. Massaging the feet at bedtime therefore helps balance prana, relax the nervous system, increase circulation, detox the body, and even relieve the day's aches and pains. A foot massage before bedtime allows you to switch off from the day and enter into a mild trance. I suspect that it supports the production of the sleep hormone melatonin to ease you into a peaceful slumber.

The Prep

Once again, feel free to use sesame oil or any other light oil for this purpose. Keep bedtime socks and a towel by your bedside to wipe off excesses.

THE PRACTICE

Wash your feet before you get into bed each night. Then massage the soles of your feet in bed before you turn the lights out.

Feel free to massage in any direction and with the pressure that you enjoy. I like long strokes and circular strokes, depending on the area. You do you; trust your body because it already knows.

Wipe off any excess oil with a towel and put on some socks before you switch off the lights.

The Dilemma

Socks at nighttime
If socks aren't your thing at bedtime, you don't need to wear them. Just ensure that all excess oil is wiped off so you don't soil your sheets.

GRATITUDE AND RADICAL ACCEPTANCE

The Wisdom

To me, gratitude is the warmest and most moist feeling in the world, and you can find more ideas on invoking feelings of gratitude in the Toolkit chapter on page 131.

However, I understand it's sometimes hard to invoke gratitude, especially when certain areas of your life feel stuck. This is where radical acceptance comes into play. When we can radically accept those areas of our lives that we have little control over or cannot change, we free up significant creative energy and space to invite in something more fulfilling and, perhaps, even start discovering our purpose in life.

For several years after moving to the US, I felt like I was caught in a headlock. I fantasized about moving back to India and took trips back to see my family at every opportunity. It was only when I could radically accept that I lived in a country far away from my family and parents that I began to thrive here.

Similarly, I carried an underlying worry about my elder daughter's endless drive and focus, afraid that she could burn out. I began imposing lunar elements on her life, which she strongly resisted. As a result, even more heat was created. Only when I could radically accept that her drive is her destiny, could I ease into our current reality and become a witness to her powerful and incredible journey. This naturally built more trust, and I became her safe place and the lunar element she was missing. When she's had an intense day, she now comes to me for a long embrace and quickly feels recharged. I occasionally top it up with a foot massage and running my hands through her hair.

I had my biggest breakthrough when I could radically accept where the world was heading, whether it was global warming, fresh potential for war, the rise of mental health disorders, or the emergence of new diseases. In the Vedas, this era is called the *Kalyug*, the era of great destruction. Instead of complaining about where we are heading and worrying about the future, I turned inward to what I called inner activism. I began focusing on the state of my world inside, instead of the unpredictable world outside. This alone expedited my healing, and you'll see that healing is contagious. When a woman heals, the whole family heals. When whole families heal, communities heal. And when communities heal, the world heals.

I have also had to radically accept things I disliked about myself. I am not the singer I wish I was. I have radically accepted that I love my occasional chai, and radically accepting it allows me to drink it without shame. Even though I teach balance to the world, I can have moments of intense imbalance, but I am on the path to progress. There are many more instances where I've had to radically accept situations, but you get what I mean.

The Prep

For this practice, you'll need an open heart and mind, and a little time in which to take yourself off to a nature spot outdoors where you won't be disturbed.

THE PRACTICE

Write down five areas of your life that you want to radically accept. They could be related to anything: your relationships, work, personal life or even the world at large. Think about each one and how they make you feel inside. Perhaps hot and dry, like an internal rush? Pick just one area that you feel the need to radically accept. Start with a relatively easy one rather than the most intense issue.

Now find some time today to go into nature. Pick up a small stone, leaf, or twig, and let it symbolize the issue you've chosen to radically accept.

Hold it between your palms and close your eyes. Now say to yourself, "I have chosen to radically accept [X]. Whenever this comes up for me, I will come to a warm and moist place within myself."

Next say, "I surrender this to the Earth, the planet, and the universe. The universe has a plan." Release the object and let it return to the Earth. If you want to take this further, dig up a little dirt, place the object there and cover it up. It's not your responsibility anymore – the universe has it covered.

Once you've enjoyed the benefits of the acceptance and healing this practice brings, find another area that requires radical acceptance and repeat the exercise all over again in a few weeks' or months' time.

The Dilemmas

Act, then surrender

Does radically accepting something mean that you're complacent about the changes your life deserves? That can be the case, especially when you've not done your part. For example, you may like to binge-watch TV late into the night, which may make you feel ashamed the next day. Radically accepting the behavior and letting the late-night binge-watch continue would be using this prompt incorrectly.

The radical acceptance here would concern the time you've wasted so far in this activity, allowing you to release the energy that was trapped in disappointment with yourself. Once you've done that, you can use the freed energy to make real change.

Radical acceptance is when you've played your part and accepted what is not in your control. But let's say that your partner's chewing noises were the reason for your daily dinner-time disharmony; radically accepting their inability to change could free up energy for both of you. Radical acceptance forces you to work on your inner world and heal from trigger patterns, rather than expending your energy on outside problems.

PART 4
AYURVEDA FOR LIFE

If you've gone deep into this book and begun to connect the dots, you may have wondered how applying the principles might change with the changing phases of life or even the seasons. Life phases and seasons are nothing but manifestations of the three inevitable cycles in the universe: growth, transformation, and decline. Each one brings a unique climate that can propel significant shifts in the body and mind. Childhood for humans and spring in the seasons are both growth phases, marked by rapid proliferation and a damp, wet climate. Adolescence and summer are when things get hotter and move towards transformation, and finally, the decline is always accompanied by the dryness of autumn or fall in mid-life, and depletion, whether it's winter or old age. Understanding and navigating through these phases is important if we want to keep our Inner Climate® warm and moist through these different stages and ages.

This section is divided into three chapters. The first will help you to make a sustainable plan for life-long mastery of the principles, while the second will enable you to understand the changes that emerge in our bodies as seasonal shifts occur on our planet. The third will help you understand your Inner Climate's® evolution as you get older so you can navigate your life more effectively as the years go by and your body ages.

YOUR PLAN FOR LIFE-LONG MASTERY

You've just experienced three weeks of intentional, intuitive living. If you've done this mindfully, you've probably connected deeply with yourself and the world around you. You may have experienced breakthroughs in some areas, while others may need a little more work. Either way, the goal of this mastery phase is to build a sustainable plan that will help you to stay on the path.

I don't want you to think of this program as something you do for just 21 days and then return back to your chaotic world. I want you to think of it as the start of the reprogramming of your entire life. Daily discoveries, periodic breakthroughs, awe and wonder, better relationships, and health will become your eternal reality. Practicing the three principles and even just bringing them to all the core areas of your life, as you have in the past 21 days, is enough. You will build a life that is better than that had by most in the world – better than your neighbor who wakes up at 4.30am to go for a run and then eats supplements for lunch, or the friend who reads every product label under a microscope but hates the world, or the billionaire who spends millions of dollars trying to live forever but lives each day in the fear of death. These 21 days will help you conquer the biggest battles and eliminate the need to fight much else.

The benefits you experience will only grow as time progresses. Take my client Nour as an example: Nour had struggled with migraines for years, and they rendered her completely dysfunctional for six days of each month. Despite trying multiple therapies for the last 10 years, she saw little to no progress. Yet her migraines became much milder when she tried reconfiguring her life over the 21 days of the healing program, which I guided her through as part of a small group. Then, within three months of living this way consistently, her migraines disappeared nearly altogether. She wrote to me expressing her disbelief. From taking at least six painkillers a month, she had now gone down to one.

As another example, Paro was on the other side of menopause and an Ayurvedic practitioner herself when I met her. She was not fully satisfied with her conventional Ayurvedic education and sought personal healing as well. Despite being on two blood pressure medications, her readings wouldn't go below 130/90. After multiple attempts to bring it down, her medical entourage accepted it as "her normal." When she saw her readings come down to 120/80 in 21 days, she was eager to share this with me, saying, "I can't believe that this is all it took."

Like Nour and Paro, I want you to stay connected to this universe's wisdom and tap into what your body already knows. These 21 days were just a glimpse into what's possible for you.

Yet, I acknowledge that these 21 days could feel really foreign for you, and you don't feel ready to bring all these changes together yet. This is where the mastery comes in. Through these prompts, you can make changes slowly, enjoying their benefits in a sustainable manner until you feel inclined to build on them and add more. I want you to be able to plan for busy days, vacations, and weekends.

YOUR STEPS TO MASTERY

Review: Turn to the Review table on page 294 in Appendix 2. You can use this as a template.

Think about each practice, one at a time. In the table, write down the benefits you experienced in the first column, the challenges in the second, and any other notes in the third.

Planning: Here's the good news. You don't have to commit to every practice. I want you to be realistic with every practice and commit only to what you can sustain. Use the Mastery table on page 296 in Appendix 2 to plan out your mastery phase.

For each practice, mark a tick or a cross in the first column, indicating whether it's a practice you're ready to bring into your life. (The ones marked with an asterisk are the bare minimum and non-negotiable if you want to see real change, but you can play about with their frequency.)

In the second column, become realistic about how many times a week you can commit to the practice, and how many minutes when applicable. Do the same for the weekend.

Here's something to think about: To keep our daily rituals alive, we may need different versions of them for different days. One of the biggest reasons people give up is because of an "all or nothing" mindset. But let's face it, life can be a wild ride – full of surprises, sudden curveballs, and moments that demand our full attention. When life gets hectic, the program can slip out of our grasp, and with this comes guilt, self-doubt, and a drop in motivation. But here's the trick: By having mini versions of our rituals in place for those chaotic days (or vacations), we still get our self-care in, keep our promises to ourselves, and avoid the guilt of falling off track. It's about working with life, not against it!

Getting back to this exercise, let's think about vacations: What rules are you going to bend? For example, before I go on vacation, I like to think ahead and modify what rules I plan to keep. On less demanding trips, I plan to exercise daily, drink warm beverages, and finish dinner by 6pm. During other trips, I may only exercise for five to seven minutes and skip all my other morning routines, but keep to my regime of cooked foods, early dinner, and warm beverages. Feel free to customize your regime according to the type of trip or vacation you're planning.

Finally, you could be in the middle of an intensely busy period. My suggestion for this one would be to shorten each routine. Plan for it in the last column. For example, let's say you exercise for 40 minutes six days a week. Your "Times a week column" could be 6d (with "d" standing for "days"), 40m (with "m" standing for "minutes"). But for intensely busy periods, I may choose 5d, 5m. Make it yours and play with it. Continue to visit it periodically to modify it according to your experiences.

I'm so excited for you to continue mastering your body, your mind, and your life. I want you to tap in to the patterns of the universe and use them to learn about your own patterns. I want you to radically accept any areas of your life that you cannot change. I want you to stay on the up instead of getting stuck in shame whenever you deviate from the path. And more than anything, I want you to tap in to what your body already knows.

THE SEASONS OF THE YEAR

I constantly marvel at how animals change their behaviors with the changing seasons. The arctic tern migrates from the Arctic to the Antarctic each year according to the seasons; bears and hedgehogs hibernate in the winter to conserve energy, and certain deer species mate at a time that ensures their offspring are born only in spring. Not only that, certain birds molt their feathers according to the weather, and other animals store food in preparation for the changing seasons. Yet somehow we humans have become so obsessed with standardizing our lives that we've forgotten to pause and acknowledge the shifts that emerge in our bodies as the seasons change. Unfortunately, our temperature-controlled environments have only furthered our negligence.

Just like the bear, deer, and the arctic tern, our bodies undergo significant shifts with the changing seasons. These changes are a result of the altering distance and exposure of our planet to the sun and moon as the Earth revolves around the sun, bringing with it climatic shifts.

While it may seem a little counterintuitive, we're going to start with the season of winter, when the Agni stokes hunger, which will help to make sense of the approaches in the seasons that follow.

Winter

Even though winter is the end of the year and a time for dryness and destruction outside, human bodies are designed for preservation during winter. Unlike the 365-day building, transformation, and decline cycle that most non-evergreen plant life follows, our cycle extends over a lifetime. Ayurvedic texts state that as the outside air cools down, the body's pores that serve as vents constrict, and the body's thermoregulation mechanism strengthens. Fluids and mucus condense in the channels of the body and become a silo – acting like an airtight container – to preserve the heat in the gut, giving rise to a strong winter hunger and a more active Agni. Our bodies are designed remarkably. Our insides are kept warm even though the air outside is chilly.

From a biological perspective, the body increases production of brown adipose tissue in the body, which is known for generating heat. The thyroid gland also ramps up the production of thyroid to increase metabolic activity.

Diet

The higher level of Agni naturally brings with it a ravenous appetite, so we can eat and digest more grounding foods and fats to help the body stay warmer. Moreover, before the invention of electricity, people had a shorter daytime window for food consumption. A high Agni ensured sufficient calories were consumed in the shorter daylight hours. Stews and broths were reserved for after dark.

You therefore want your winter menus to include good fats, whole grains, root vegetables, milk proteins, warming spices, nuts, and seeds. Despite being a fruit lover, I take a complete break from fruit for the three winter months, which are December, January, and February in the Northern Hemisphere and June, July, and August in the Southern Hemisphere. Doing winter right keeps spring allergies and flu at bay.

Winter is the worst time to go on a diet or long fast; if the strong Agni remains unfed, it will eat up softer tissues. But it's the best time to celebrate food, as your digestion is at its best.

Even though the sunset is earlier, this is the time when your endogenous clock (body clock) trumps the exogenous (sun clock), and you can continue to eat your light dinner at your regular time or slightly earlier, by 30 to 60 minutes.

Exercise

Since we don't sweat much in the winter, electrolytes are preserved in the body, and it doesn't tire easily, making this the ideal time to exercise. At the same time, the Inner Climate® and body fluids are already dense, so exercise will help to melt and soften things rather than allow the winter to cause dryness. If there is one time in the year you can be a bit more intense with your exercise routine, it's winter. If you recall, the first rule of exercise is to consume good fats when actively exercising; again, easy in the winter.

Sleep

Plan to go to sleep slightly earlier and for longer during the winter months. While humans don't hibernate during the winter, I suspect our ancestors spent a good chunk of their 24-hour winter days in relative hibernation compared to other seasons. Sleep allows the body to stay grounded and warm, protecting it against the harsh winter.

Other winter rituals include massaging your body with oil, dry massaging with thumps to loosen fluids, and the use of musk, which is currently being explored for its use in depression. I suspect that Ayurveda advocated its use in fighting winter depression as the serotonin levels that contribute to a good mood naturally decline at this time of year.

Spring

As winter ends, the sun's rays become sharper and begin to melt everything that was frozen. This applies not only to the snow and ice but to the fluids and mucus in our body, which have thickened during the winter. As a result, the body is now overflowing with sticky, melting mucus that attracts pollen and other allergens. It doesn't matter what your Inner Climate® is, it will become less dry and more humid in the spring. If you usually have a dry Inner Climate®, you may enjoy this new moisture. And remarkably, spring is known to be a time for peak fertility for many species, including humans. However, if you are already humid, you could experience spring sluggishness and perhaps even colds, flus, and allergies now.

Diet

The body thermoregulates and perspires as the Earth warms up outside, and the vents of the body and its pores expand. The warm silo effect that was created for the Agni due to the constricted pores and dense fluids no longer exists. As a result, the Agni weakens, and the body has to undergo drastic shifts, making it vulnerable to many diseases.

The Ayurvedic texts recommend a lighter and drier diet in the spring. Spring foods include roasted flour, barley, drier seasonal vegetables, honey, and barbecues. Fruits should be introduced slowly to the diet as they can aggravate mucus production, especially during early spring. Experiment with fruit during the daytime and notice if it makes you sniffle more. Then gradually increase your intake from there, reserving consumption for daytime only.

You can infuse your water with honey if you drink it at room temperature, or with dried ginger if you drink it warm or hot. Honey helps to absorb and dry out excess mucus from the body. The caveat is that honey cannot be warmed or consumed in anything hotter than a lukewarm temperature, as it can create toxicity in the body. In fact, research is now being done to examine the toxicity of a compound called hydroxy-methylfurfural, which is generated when honey is heated.[9]

Exercise

The body can tire a little more easily in the spring, releasing excess bodily fluids through sweat. Thus, while exercise is important at this time of year, it can be at slightly less intense levels than in winter.

Sleep

Spring afternoons can bring sluggishness. After all, mucus doesn't allow for ease of breathing and, as a result, affects oxygen intake and the overall state of the body. Unfortunately, sleeping in the afternoons will further perpetuate the problem. After all, sleeping is lunar and when done in the daytime, it slows bodily function. However, exercising every day to release fluids will make nighttime sleep easier during spring by reducing congestion in the body.

Summer

With the arrival of summer, everything becomes drier – the ground, the air, and the human body. The body's pores are wide open and electrolytes are lost through perspiration. By the end of the summer, the Earth often becomes parched, ready for the fall.

Diet

The Agni is at its weakest and the body experiences a reduced appetite but an increased thirst during the summer. At this time of year, the body craves sour-tasting drinks, as sourness feels refreshing and instantly triggers our appetite. (Refer to the section on summer drinks in Day 11, "Regulate Your Water Consumption," in Part 3.) The summer diet is meant to be lighter and more refreshing than at other times of year, with generous quantities of watery foods like soups, broths, and rice congee. White rice is recommended for its innate cooling properties.

Due to its intensity, the sun precooks many foods like fruits; after all, this is the season of transformation. It's the best time to enjoy fruits and certain vegetables like cucumbers. No matter what the season, fruits are best consumed during the daytime between the hours of 10am and 4pm. Eating fruit early in the morning will prevent the body from getting fired up and ready for the day. After 4pm, the Agni is actively declining, and breaking down sweet and mushy fruit would further diminish its strength. I love my fruits, but I like to consume them as a mid-morning snack around 10.30am or as a mid-afternoon snack around 3pm. Like I mentioned before, I avoid most fresh fruits altogether in the months of December, January, and February, when my pantry gets loaded with dried fruits and nuts instead.

Exercise

Heavy exercise is contraindicated during summer as the body is already depleted. In fact, exercise is completely contraindicated during the hottest days. I recommend light yoga for most of the summer. Going too intense during the summer months could deplete the body of essential moisture and make your Inner Climate® drier. This is also one reason many people see an increase in hair loss by the end of summer.

Sleep

The good news is that daytime napping, which is contraindicated during other months, is allowed during the hottest summer days to preserve moisture; thus the summer siesta. Given the longer summer days, taking a nap also allows for a slightly later bedtime.

Fall

The fall is the time of year when the warmth and transformation of the summer months begin to give way to the chill, crisp winds of autumn, when flowers fade and leaves wither and turn to gold. Fruits can be enjoyed till early fall; I always recommend cooking apples and pears once this season is at its peak. Our bodies are beginning to ready themselves now for winter, slowing down.

Think of the fall as being a sweet transition period between summer and winter, where you can slowly ease into winter-time grounding recommendations and adapt your approach to your diet, exercise, and sleep accordingly with this time of gentle change.

Living with the Seasons

Adjusting your lifestyle and diet according to the seasons can really help to lower the load on the immune system and improve your overall well-being.

Zuma's daughters, Mia (19) and Mila (17), suffered from severe spring allergies and had been relying upon allergy medication to get through March and April since their early teens. Zuma had recently gotten into alternative and more holistic therapies for her third daughter, who suffered from an idiopathic condition. Upon seeing the benefits, she was now open to considering Ayurveda for her first two as well.

When Zuma first came to see me with her girls in March, I gave them some herbs but insisted that they came back later in the year, in November, as preparation for spring begins during the fall. When I saw her daughters' food journals, I was sad but not shocked. Instead of taking advantage of the winter Agni, these girls had been drinking frozen fruit smoothies in the colder months to get their bodies ready for spring and summer. Not only that, but Mila suffered from chronic bloating and mild tummy ache, which only got worse as the year became warmer. Her gut wasn't warm and moist, nor was it her friend.

They returned to see me that same November. It took some convincing to get the sisters to replace their smoothies with soups, and they initially refused to add other calorie-rich foods during the winter at first. Soon enough, they experienced better energy levels and Mila noticed a significant shift in her bloat. In a month's time, they were willing to go all warm and even to add some whole grains and root vegetables to their diet.

When spring arrived, their allergies did return but were significantly milder than in the previous years. They now used allergy medication as needed instead of using it as a daily survival tool. I'm certain that as Mia and Mila continue to follow their seasonal regimens, they'll not only experience an allergy-free spring, but also an improved relationship with their food and better moods.

If you live in a place where the seasons are not quite similar to the ones described above, use your newly developed insight to determine the state of your local climate, your Agni and your perspiration levels, and thus the needs of your body from season to season, and modify your diet and lifestyle accordingly (see Appendix 4: "Seasons". Page 299).

THE SEASONS OF LIFE

Climate and landscape shifts go hand in hand, in the world outside us and the world inside. As the body's landscape changes through the phases of life, so does its climate – and vice versa, as my friend Trevor was to experience first-hand.

Trevor was a gym instructor and a nutritionist, who helped women build more muscle mass. I met him on a flight from LA to NYC and we found we had a lot to agree and disagree on during the course of our five-and-a-half-hour journey. He had primarily looked at Eastern sciences like Ayurveda as being "woo-woo" but was happy to listen to my perspectives.

He leaned in closer to listen when I talked about metabolic changes in women as we age and our inability to digest large amounts of proteins during the menopause years and after. He confessed that even his most conscious clients in that age range suffered from severe bloating and discomfort from the same foods that his 20- to 30-year-olds could digest with more ease. Additionally, even though he hadn't thought about it earlier, he was able to relate to the drying of the skin and body as we age.

I knew I'd stirred something in him when he called me the following week, interested to learn more about abhyanga and its benefits. For the next six months, Trevor systemically worked with me to understand Ayurvedic nutrition principles for women of different ages. Even though he didn't take every leaf out of my book, he was able to absorb some core principles for use with his clients and felt very happy with the result.

Trevor and I became friends and a couple of years later, he jokingly introduced me to one of his clients as "the person who helped him help his clients age like wine." However, the fact is that Ayurveda can help us at any time of life, as long as we understand the climatic shifts happening in our body from the spring of childhood to the winter of old age.

Childhood – the Spring of Life

Childhood is the growth phase, aka the spring of life, and the body's condition is much like that of spring: wet but even more tender, like soil that has seen its first harvest. During this time, growth hormone is at its highest and the body's climate is juicy, so new cells can be generated quickly. The Agni is absent at birth as breastmilk is predigested and gradually builds up as the microbiome passes from the breastmilk into the baby's body. With limited gut flora, a child's body is vulnerable until it can gradually gain heat and strength.

Diet

The basic dietary principle for growing children is light, nourishing, and warm. Moderate amounts of building foods such as rice, almonds, ghee, and fleshy vegetables are essential. However, when it comes to young children, a little food goes a long way; it's a misconception that children must be overfed in these growing years. During these years, the body is very effective in using food to generate energy and nutrients. Since the Agni is still not at its full power, overfeeding can lead to discomfort and indigestion. I see this as being one of the main causes of illness in children who get sick repeatedly.

Certain foods are especially harmful during this phase. While children are naturally attracted to sweet-tasting foods, processed foods and refined sugar can dampen the already wet body, making it a breeding ground for parasites. Similarly, cold beverages make it harder for the gut to remain warm and moist.

I'm reminded of the case of Jonah, a seven-year-old who loved football and who was desperate to play for his local junior side during the fall season. But the coach had mandated that players had to have an 80 percent school attendance rate, and his mother, Kelsey, was concerned as Jonah had missed significant amounts of school due to his congestion and subsequent lack of energy.

Kelsey was certainly more conscientious than many parents I've met. She shopped only at the farmers' market, didn't use a microwave and cooked fresh produce for Jonah several times a week. She blamed his lack of immunity on something more innate. However, I was soon to discover that the real trouble lay with the milk he'd been drinking three times a day, of which at least one glass was organic but cold chocolate milk. Since Jonah's schedule was rammed with classes, his mother found this to be the most effective way of feeding him well.

We stopped all his dairy at first; I knew from experience that switching from cold to warm milk was a mighty task. When Kelsey noticed that Jonah had been well for three weeks in a row, she was willing to give warm milk a shot. We started with a tepid cup of hot chocolate. Eventually, Jonah was able to manage two cups of hot milk a day, one with chocolate and one infused with turmeric. He still had occasional bouts of sickness, as most kids do, but his congestion and repeated colds were now gone.

Another taste that children find tricky is bitterness. If you're a parent, you'll know that kids are overly sensitive to, and detest anything, bitter. Well, children's palates are designed to reject bitter foods, as these are generally scraping and not as nourishing for the system. So, my suggestion is to keep those bitter foods out of their diet till their palate naturally begins to accept them during adolescence and their late teens.

When Suhani, my eldest, was eight years old, we went out for lunch with her feisty classmate, Zina. Zina had dry, flaky eczema all over her face and was constantly itching. My curiosity got the better of me when Zina passed on the French fries and pizza, and instead asked if we could order an arugula (rocket) apple salad for lunch.

"Do you like salads, Zina?" I asked.

"I love salads, and my mom said that they're good for me," she said and seemed genuinely excited.

While there can be other underlying causes for her eczema, I was certain that bitter dry salads didn't help. So many parents use adult nutrition principles for their children in a very well-intentioned manner, but end up causing more damage instead. If you are a parent, I suggest you read this chapter twice and really think about its meaning and application. What does it mean for your child or children? What changes will you make?

Exercise

Exercise can be tricky for children, especially when it builds too much muscle. Muscle, by design, is tight and stiff, and reduces the body's ability to stretch and grow lengthwise. Similarly, exercises like yoga that require a lot of stretching and varied poses should be undertaken with great care by children, as their bones are still malleable at that age. My personal belief is that children need movement more than exercise, and sports offer a great solution.

Sleep

Children have high amounts of growth hormone to support their rapid increase in size. As we've seen, during the 24-hour period, the levels of growth hormone are at their highest in deep sleep, in the dead of the night; thus a good night's sleep is essential for growth. Additionally, the nervous system is very tender and constantly processing new information and making new connections. Sleep allows the nervous system to rest and internalize these new connections.

In the years leading up to adolescence, the body starts to warm up with the onset of hormones. This newly ignited fire explains why teens suddenly develop a mind of their own. Once teens reach adult height, the Agni is stabilized, and they are officially in the summer of their lives.

Youth – the Summer of Life

Youth is the transformation phase or summer of life. Estrogen and progesterone, the two beautiful female hormones, come into play and create warmth during this time. Estrogen is primarily responsible for the development of secondary sexual characteristics, bone growth, and regulation of the menstrual cycles, while progesterone prepares the body for a potential pregnancy.

Adolescence can be compared to an oil lamp filled with oil to the brim. Full of fuel, as we go through the years of our youth, we keep burning through the oil until it is depleted, the flame burns down, and we enter the dry phase of life. Doing adolescence and youth right means preserving this fuel so that the body can keep everything warm and moist for longer. It means playing the long-term game rather than burning out too quickly.

However, our lifestyles today are quite the opposite. Our overly solar ways of living mean that we burn too fiercely and deplete our juices. Over-productivity, excess exercise, low-fat foods, caffeine, alcohol, and late nights expedite our journey to the dry side. This is also a leading cause of infertility, as moisture is key for conception.

My recommendation for the youthful years would therefore be to balance solar with lunar energies consistently and constantly, and to focus on nourishing the body and the mind. Most of the ideas in this book aim to support and sustain the fertile conditions of these years.

Diet

As we have seen throughout this book, a balanced diet full of good fats and spices will support the sort of good health and vitality that we associate with the youthful summer years of life. Eating well and at the appropriate times of day can help to keep the inner flame fueled with good oils and the Agni burning brightly. For a reminder of the key dietary principles, revisit the chapter on the gut and your diet in Part 2, and dip into Days 1, 2, 3, 4, 5, and 12 in Part 3.

Exercise

If you wish to retain the vitality of youth, exercise is important. Do your chosen form of exercise between 6am and 10am, making sure your diet includes plenty of good fats. Remember to choose an activity that suits your own Inner Climate®, and exercise to half your capacity in any single session. For a recap on other general principles, turn to the chapter on exercise in Part 2 and Day 8 in Part 3.

Sleep

As we've seen, exercise is a solar activity that needs to be balanced with the lunar qualities of sleep. Sleep, oil massage, meditation, rest, silent time, and phone-free times are all essential if we want to slow down our decline into dryness. For a reminder of the key steps needed for a good night's sleep, turn to the chapter on sleep in Part 2 and Day 10 in Part 3.

Middle Age – the Fall of Life

As the transformation phase nears its end, the body starts to dry up. When we reach the autumn or fall years of life, the oil in our lamp likewise begins to run dry. For a short while, the body's inner flame may burn more brightly as it begins to run out of fuel before it completely extinguishes itself. Estrogen and progesterone levels begin to fluctuate in the body before their eventual decline, affecting overall moisture, moods, menstrual cycles, and more. Perimenopausal women can also experience this as hot flashes that will eventually settle down. This may be the time of life in which we are on the other side of the pinnacle of our careers, and we start to consider slowing down and making plans for retirement. However, we will still benefit from the advice mapped out in Part 3, "Your 21-Day Healing Program."

Diet

As the flame of the Agni naturally begins to dwindle at this time of life, we may find that we need to consume fewer calories, or we will begin to put on weight. In this drier and cooler life season, look at introducing moderate helpings of warm and moist foods like avocados, sweet potatoes, zucchini (courgette), squashes, cooked grains, coconuts, and ghee into your diet. I also want you to think of oil massage as an important part of your diet in this phase. After all, your skin is a channel of consumption and oil is its food – very nourishing indeed, without the calories.

Exercise

Exercising during these years can become difficult due to aching joints and excess weight, but is absolutely essential for maintaining long-term mobility and health. A yoga routine that combines flexibility and strength is ideal. For cardio, my favorite is taking a gentle cardio dance class and then building it up. Dancing is an exercise not only for the body but also for the mind. Here too, whatever exercise you choose to do, abhayanga or oil massage is great to protect your joints and support your muscles.

Sleep

Sleep can become a challenge for many women during this phase of life, as the body is gradually losing its lunar juices. However, meditation and pranayama and other deep relaxation techniques can serve as a great substitute in enabling the type of important repair work in the body that would otherwise come with slumber. Different studies have shown that an hour of meditation may amount to anywhere from one to four hours of nighttime sleep. Start with a short five-minute meditation practice and then gradually increase this to 7, 10, 15, 20, 30, 45, and eventually 60 minutes. You'll be surprised with how much easier it becomes to sit longer when you build it up gradually.

One thing I must warn you here is that lack of nighttime sleep can result in daytime sluggishness, and I come across many women in this phase of life who resort to daytime napping. Not only will this hurt your metabolic juices but it will worsen the problem of your nighttime sleep. At the same time, less sleep time at night may sometimes mean more screen time, and screen time will only dry your eyes and frazzle your nerves even further. My suggestion would be to become mindful that sleep may be lighter and shorter and find solace in your meditation practice and more grounding hobbies.

Old Age – the Winter of Life

The oil in our lamp has now run dry, the flame dims, and the body likewise becomes dry and cold. Estrogen and progesterone have stabilized at significantly lower levels. In fact, this can be a time (post-menopause) for great self-discovery, especially for women, many of whom may find themselves removed from the dating, mating, and nesting game for the very first time.

Caring for this phase of life means bringing in moisture in other ways, such as through oil massages, sleep, and meditation.

Diet

As the oil lamp loses its heat, so does the Agni. Many women in their fifties and sixties complain of bloating and indigestion. I therefore recommend reducing dinner to a light broth and reducing food quantities by 30 percent. Dates, maca root extract, almonds, rice, and soups are especially nourishing and grounding for the earlier decades of this season of life.

Additionally, since the body is losing heat and thus the ability to break down fats and heavy foods, I recommend lowering fat and protein levels to a level that the body can digest.

Exercise

In the winter years of life, our joints can start to stiffen up, which is when we will benefit from activities such as Pilates, yoga, stretch classes, and gentle outings in nature. Running can become detrimental at this age as the physical impact can lead to rapid dryness, depletion, and excess pressure on the joints. So if you are a runner, consider taking brisk walks instead.

Another thing to note during these years is that the bone marrow can start to become drier, which means that abhyanga becomes even more critical if you're exercising. Oiling the navel daily with three to four drops can also support the Agni and metabolic strength.

Navel oiling, an ancient Ayurvedic practice, is suitable for people of all ages, including babies. Although the belly button served as the center for nourishment in the womb via the umbilical cord, it is often overlooked after birth.

In an Ayurvedic practice known as the pechoti method, warm oil is applied to the navel, which is connected to thousands of nerves, making it an effective point for absorbing the healing properties of oils. This practice is believed to enhance digestion, balance hormones, hydrate the skin, relieve joint and muscle pain, support detoxification, and improve emotional well-being. To practice, choose an oil like sesame, coconut, almond, or castor oil, gently warm it, and apply 5 to 10 drops to the navel while lying down. Massage the area in gentle circular motions and let the oil absorb for 10 to 15 minutes, ideally before bed.

Sleep

Sleep may become more elusive during this time, but this is an invitation to deepen your meditation practice, perhaps even embracing the quiet stillness of the early morning. Reflect on your journey: Who do you need to forgive? What burdens are you ready to release? What holds your heart to this body and life, even as it begins its gentle descent? As you move into your seventies and eighties, start preparing your mind for the moment when you will eventually let go (see Appendix 5: "Life Seasons". Page 300). At the age of 42, I've already begun this practice. It may sound unsettling, but it's deeply freeing. It makes me want to live more fully. I imagine myself weightless, unburdened, my heart overflowing with gratitude for the life I've lived, without a trace of regret – ready to surrender into the unknown, not with fear, but with peace.

On a lighter note, napping for a few minutes (around 20 to 40 minutes) is completely acceptable for most in their seventies and above, so if that's you, enjoy your siesta!

CONCLUSION

As I bring this book to a close, my heart overflows with gratitude and fulfillment. Within these pages, I've shared the timeless wisdom handed down from my ancestors, the profound teachings of Ayurveda, and the insights from my own healing journey. These principles have not only enriched my life day by day over the last few decades but have also brought me to a place of greater strength and happiness at the age of 42 than I ever knew at 21.

Living in the heart of New York City with two teenage daughters, I don't wear the robes of a monk, yet I've found a peace that rivals that of any monastery. These teachings have allowed me to engage fully with the world without being ensnared by it. I continue to heal and grow inwardly, even as my body gracefully moves through the natural process of aging. Most days, I sleep deeply and peacefully, my body free from aches, my cycles still in harmony. I savor life's simple pleasures – samosas, kettle-cooked chips – and dance with abandon in the city I love.

This sense of freedom and well-being is not exclusive to me. You, too, can experience the boundless vitality and joy that comes from true wellness, rather than living in fear of illness.

Thank you for trusting me to be the vessel of this profound knowledge. My hope is that you immerse yourself in these teachings, read this book again, and allow it to transform your life as it has for so many others. The path to well-being is yours to walk, and the freedom it brings is within your reach.

APPENDIX 1
MENU OPTIONS AND RECIPES

Menu Options

Breakfast

Options:
- Hot raab (sweet or savory malt drink)
- Steel-cut oatmeal porridge
- Stewed apples
- Roasted sweet potatoes
- Hot spiced milk with almonds

Lunch

Options:
- Grain and lentil bowl with veggies
- Ayurvedic mujadara
- Mexican rice with black beans
- Ayurvedic kitchari with buttermilk
- Ayurvedic pilaf with yogurt dip

Dinner

Options:
- Mung lentil stew
- Ayurvedic chickpea and veggie stew
- Simple barley stew
- Favorite vegetable stew
- Simple spiced vegetable soup, served with a side of veggies, rice, or a small piece of warmed sourdough with olive oil

Bedtime beverage: Hot raab (sweet or savory malt drink)

Recipes

All recipes serve two to three people, unless otherwise stated.

Before diving into the recipes, I want to address a common misconception about Ayurveda and its stance on onions, garlic, and meat. It's often believed that Ayurveda outright condemns these, but that's not historically accurate. Ayurveda embraces whatever tools it can to restore balance and harmony in the body's Inner Climate®. Here's a deeper perspective ...

Meat

While I am passionately plant-based, with the exception of dairy for ghee, milk, and yogurt, Ayurveda has historically utilized bone broths and meat soups, especially for those suffering from a cold, dry, or depleted Inner Climate®. However, the modern state of animal farming raises concerns for me. Animals today live in chronic states of fear, their bodies flooded with stress hormones and injected with growth enhancers. These conditions permeate the meat, contributing to inflammation and imbalances when consumed. That said, I recognize that the choice to consume meat is deeply personal, and each individual must decide what feels right for them.

Garlic and Onions

Many who approach Ayurveda through the lens of yoga choose to avoid garlic and onions, and there's wisdom in this practice. Yoga's path seeks calm, clarity, and detachment from worldly distractions. Garlic and onions, known to stimulate the nervous system and heat the body, are believed to intensify passion and disrupt the meditative state. For the yogi, who values stillness and focus, these foods may pose challenges by pulling the mind outward rather than allowing it to turn inward.

Garlic, with its heating quality, can actually support the breakdown of cholesterol-related plaque and help clear excess phlegm from the body. Personally, I enjoy using both garlic and onions for their flavor and health benefits. However, I must admit that when I visit my paternal home, where they abstain from using anything that grows below the ground, I involuntarily refrain from garlic and onions. During those times, I notice a unique sense of calm and clarity that arises – a subtle yet profound shift in my inner state.

Ayurveda, at its core, respects individual choices and personal needs. It offers guidance, but it's up to you to decide what works best for your body and inner state.

Sweet Raab

Raab (malt drink) is typically enjoyed warm and can be a great comfort drink, especially during colder months. It's a completely nourishing meal and can be a substitute for hot chocolate.

Prep time: 5 minutes
Cook time: 25 minutes
Serves 4

Ingredients

2 tablespoons ghee (clarified butter)
2 tablespoons millet flour (either pearl or foxtail) or whole-wheat flour
2 cups (17fl oz/500ml) water
½ teaspoon ground ginger
½ teaspoon ground cardamom (optional)
2 cups (17fl oz/500ml) whole milk (A2, organic, grass-fed is best)
1–2 tablespoons jaggery powder or brown sugar
5–7 almonds, soaked and sliced (see tip below, optional)

Method

1. In a heavy-bottomed pan, heat the ghee over medium heat.
2. Add the flour and roast until it turns golden brown and emits a pleasant aroma. This should take 5 to 7 minutes. Stir continuously with a spatula to prevent burning. Take special care to mix in any flour that may have stuck to the side of the pan.

3. Slowly add the water to the roasted flour, stirring continuously with a whisk to break down any lumps.
4. Add the ground ginger, and cardamom, if using.
5. Continue to cook the mixture on medium heat, stirring continuously until it thickens. This will take about 10 minutes.
6. Add the whole milk to the mixture and stir well.
7. Add the jaggery or sugar and mix until it dissolves completely.
8. Continue to cook for another 5 to 7 minutes, stirring occasionally, until the raab reaches a thick, creamy consistency. Remove it from the heat.
9. Pour the raab into serving glasses or bowls.
10. Garnish with sliced almonds if desired.
11. Serve hot.

Tip: Soak your almonds overnight in a little water, then peel and slice them. There are a few reasons for soaking. Firstly, soaking improves their digestibility and makes them easier to chew thoroughly. Secondly, the peel contains tannins, which can affect nutrient absorption. Also, soaking almonds overnight changes their warm potency to being cooler on the system.

Savory Malt

Savory malt or raab is typically enjoyed warm and is a great option for a nourishing and comforting drink and is usually lighter than the sweet malt. It's the perfect warm and moist choice for breakfast, especially in the winter months.

Prep time: 5 minutes
Cook time: 20 minutes
Serves 2 to 3

Ingredients

1 tablespoon ghee (clarified butter)
2 tablespoons bajra (pearl millet or another colored millet flour)
½ teaspoon cumin seeds
½ teaspoon ajwain (carom seeds)
A pinch of asafetida (hing) powder (optional)
½ teaspoon ground ginger or 1 teaspoon grated fresh ginger
¼ teaspoon turmeric powder
About 4 cups (35fl oz/1 liter) water
Salt, to taste
1–2 tablespoons yogurt (optional, for added tanginess)
Freshly ground black pepper, to taste
1 tablespoon chopped fresh cilantro (coriander) (optional)

Method

1. In a heavy-bottomed pan, heat the ghee over medium heat.
2. Add the flour and roast it until it turns golden brown and emits a pleasant aroma. This should take about 5 to 7 minutes. Stir continuously to prevent burning.

Take special care to mix in any flour that may have stuck to the side of the pan.

3. Add the cumin seeds, ajwain seeds, and asafetida to the roasted flour and sauté for a minute. You can also bloom (see page 191) these on the side and add them to the roast flour mix.

4. Add the ground ginger (or grated fresh ginger) and turmeric powder and mix well.

5. Slowly add about one-quarter of the water to the mixture and mix to make a paste. Then add the remaining water, stirring continuously to avoid lumps.

6. Add salt to taste.

7. Continue to cook the mixture on medium heat, stirring continuously until it thickens a little. This will take about 15 minutes.

8. If using, whip or mix the yogurt with some water to an even mixture and then add to the pan. Mix well to incorporate, then remove the pan from the heat.

9. Add freshly ground black pepper to taste.

10. Pour the savory raab into serving bowls.

11. Garnish with chopped fresh cilantro.

12. Serve hot.

Tip: For a thicker consistency, add less water and reduce the cooking time by a couple of minutes, or as required.

Steel-Cut Oatmeal Porridge

My 16-year-old has been eating this steel-cut porridge five days a week for over a decade and is still not bored of it. I would also recommend trying a variation where you completely eliminate the ghee and the sautéing to make a lighter version, especially if your Inner Climate® is sluggish and dense. Instead, add a teaspoon of ghee or coconut oil after the oatmeal is cooked and stir it in evenly.

Prep time: 5 minutes
Cook time: 35 minutes
Serves 2 to 3

Ingredients

½ tablespoon ghee (clarified butter)
¾ cup (3½oz/100g) steel-cut oats (coarse oatmeal)
3–4 cups (26–35fl oz/750ml–1 liter) water
1inch (2.5cm) Ceylon cinnamon stick
½ teaspoon ground cardamom
¼ teaspoon ground ginger
A pinch of ground rock salt or Himalayan pink salt
2 tablespoons raisins
2 tablespoons sliced almonds (ideally soaked overnight, peeled and sliced – see page 259)

Method

1. In a medium saucepan, heat the ghee over medium heat.
2. Add the oats and sauté for 2 to 3 minutes until they are lightly toasted and fragrant.
3. Add the water to the saucepan and bring it to a boil. Throw in the cinnamon stick.

4. Reduce the heat to low, then add the ground cardamom, ground ginger, and salt.
5. Stir well, then let the oats simmer uncovered, stirring occasionally, for about 20 to 25 minutes, or until the oats are tender and the mixture has thickened to your desired consistency.
6. Once the oats are cooked, add the raisins and sliced almonds before serving.

Stewed Apples

In my household, fresh uncooked fruit is a rarity during the colder months, but stewed apples are the perfect way to enjoy the season's final harvest. As fall winds down, this comforting dish brings warmth and nourishment while making the most of nature's bounty.

Prep time: 5 minutes
Cook time: 15 minutes
Serves 2 to 3

Ingredients

3 medium apples (preferably a sweet variety such as Fuji, Gala, or Honeycrisp)
½ tablespoon ghee (clarified butter)
1 cinnamon stick or ½ teaspoon ground cinnamon
3 to 4 whole cloves
½ cup (4fl oz/120ml) water
A pinch of ground cardamom (optional)

Method

1. Peel, core, and chop the apples into bite-sized pieces. Set aside.
2. In a medium saucepan, heat the ghee over medium heat.
3. If using a cinnamon stick, add it to the ghee and let it toast for a minute.
4. Add the cloves and toast for another 30 seconds.
5. Add the chopped apples to the saucepan and stir to coat them in the ghee and spices.
6. Add the water and bring to a gentle simmer.

7. Once the apples are stewed and tender, remove the cinnamon stick (if necessary) and cloves.
8. Stir in the ground cinnamon (if using) and a pinch of ground cardamom for extra flavor.
9. Divide the stewed apples into serving bowls.

Roasted Sweet Potatoes

One reason why sweet potatoes are so satisfying is that they are sweet and moist, just like most nourishing foods – such as rice, milk, and coconuts. But the creamy texture of the sweet potato and its health benefits for those whose Agnis are still happy are innumerable. If you like your sweet potatoes to be softer on the inside and crispier outside, boil the potatoes first, then roast them for less time in the oven.

Prep time: 5 minutes
Cook time: 30 minutes
Serves 2 to 3

Ingredients

2 medium sweet potatoes
2 tablespoons olive oil or ghee
½ teaspoon ground cumin
¼ teaspoon ground cinnamon
Salt to taste
Freshly ground black pepper, to taste
Seasoning mix of your choice (such as parsley and thyme)
Dash of lemon juice
Fresh herbs, such as parsley or cilantro (coriander), to garnish

Method

1. Preheat your oven to 425°F (220°C, gas 7).
2. Wash and peel the sweet potatoes.
3. Cut them into small, evenly-sized cubes (about 1-inch/2.5-cm pieces).
4. In a large bowl, combine the sweet potato cubes, olive oil or ghee, cumin, cinnamon, and salt.

5. Toss well to ensure the sweet potatoes are evenly coated with the oil and cumin.
6. Spread the sweet potato cubes in a single layer on a baking sheet.
7. Roast in the preheated oven for 20 minutes (if boiled first), or until the sweet potatoes are tender and slightly crispy at the edges (25-30 mins). Toss halfway through for even roasting.
8. Season the sweet potatoes with black pepper and seasoning mix.
9. Add a dash of lemon juice.
10. Transfer the potatoes to a serving dish.
11. Garnish with fresh herbs.

Hot Spiced Milk with Almonds

Milk has grown to become my comfort food, but I rarely drink it uncooked or even plain. This is a richer version of my daily cardamom milk – my morning comfort. My daughters will drink this over hot chocolate, and that speaks for itself.

Prep time: 5 minutes
Cook time: 5 minutes
Serves 1

Ingredients

A few saffron strands (optional, for added luxury and benefits)
1 cup (9fl oz/250ml) milk (preferably whole and organic)
1 teaspoon maple syrup
1 teaspoon ground cinnamon
A pinch of ground cardamom (optional, for added flavor and digestive benefits)
A pinch of turmeric powder (optional, for its anti-inflammatory properties)
1 teaspoon sliced almonds (ideally soaked overnight, peeled, and sliced)

Method

1. If you are using saffron, add the strands to a tablespoon of the milk in a small bowl and set aside to soak for 5 to 10 minutes while you work on the preparing the rest of the recipe.
2. Gently heat the milk in a saucepan over medium heat until it is hot but not boiling.
3. Stir in the maple syrup.

4. Add the cinnamon, cardamom (if using), and turmeric powder (if using). Stir well to combine.
5. Pour the warm milk into a cup and, if using, add the saffron and its soaking liquid.
6. Sprinkle the sliced almonds on top.
7. Stir well and enjoy the warm, comforting beverage.

Grain and Lentil Bowl with Veggies

A grain and lentil or bean bowl is the ideal way to bring all essential elements into one tasteful dish. This recipe aims to give you a formula to make your own bowls. A type of lentil, a grain, spiced veggies, herbs, and a balanced condiment or dressing. Et voilà!

Prep time: 10 minutes (plus soaking time for lentils)
Cook time: 30–40 minutes (depending on grains and lentils)
Serves 2 to 3

Ingredients

1 cup (6¼oz/180g) lentils of choice: mung beans, black lentils, brown lentils, red lentils, or green lentils
1 cup (6¼oz/180g) grain of your choice: rice, bulgur wheat, spelt, barley, or local millet
2 bay leaves (optional)
2 cinnamon sticks (optional)
1–1½ tablespoons ghee or extra virgin olive oil
Garlic (optional)
Spices of your choice: ground cumin, ground coriander, black pepper, thyme, oregano, Italian mixed seasoning
Veggies of choice: zucchini (courgette), squash, root vegetables, cruciferous vegetables (such as broccoli or cauliflower), or alliums (such as onions or leeks)
Condiment or sauce of your choice: e.g. pesto, hummus with olive oil, or roasted red-pepper dressing
Herbs of your choice: cilantro (coriander), basil, or parsley
Salt and black pepper, to taste

Method

1. Rinse the lentils and soak them in water for about 30 minutes to an hour.
2. Drain and rinse the soaked lentils.
3. Rinse your chosen grain under cold water.
4. Cook the grain in a saucepan according to the packet instructions. Add a bay leaf or a cinnamon stick (if using) to the cooking water. Once cooked, set aside.
5. Put the lentils in a pot with enough water to cover them. Add a bay leaf or cinnamon stick (if using). Cook until tender, about 20 to 30 minutes. Drain off any excess water, if needed, and set aside.
6. Heat the ghee or oil in a large frying pan and add the garlic, your chosen spices, and the vegetables. Sauté until well cooked.
7. In a bowl, neatly place the cooked grains, lentils, and roasted veggies, side by side.
8. Drizzle with your chosen condiment or sauce and garnish with herbs.
9. Season with salt and pepper to taste.
10. Mix everything together and enjoy warm.

Ayurvedic Mujadara

Mujadara is a classic dish made from lentils and groats (often rice) and garnished with sautéed or caramelized onions. Enjoy this warm with a side of veggies. It also pairs well with Ayurvedic Buttermilk (see page 280).

Prep time: 15 minutes (plus soaking time)
Cook time: 25–30 minutes
Serves 2 to 3

Ingredients

1 cup (6oz/170g) brown lentils
½ cup (3oz/85g) aged rice (organic sona masuri or basmati)
    or bulgur wheat
2 tablespoons ghee or olive oil
1 large onion, thinly sliced
3 cups (26fl oz/750ml) water or vegetable broth
¼ inch cinnamon stick
½ teaspoon salt (or to taste)
A squeeze of fresh lemon juice
½ teaspoon ground cumin, roasted (see page 000)
½ teaspoon sumac (optional)
Fresh cilantro (coriander) or parsley, to garnish

Method

1. Rinse the lentils under cold water, then leave to soak in a bowl of fresh water for about 30 minutes to an hour.
2. Rinse the rice or bulgur wheat, then leave to soak in a separate bowl for 20 minutes.
3. Add the ghee or olive oil to a large deep pot and place over medium heat.

4. Once hot, add the sliced onion.
5. Sauté the onion for about 15 minutes, stirring occasionally, until golden brown and caramelized, with crispy edges.
6. Remove the caramelized onion and set aside on a paper-towel-lined plate to remove any excess oil.
7. Add the rinsed and drained lentils to the same pan and cook for a few minutes. If you need more oil, add some so that the rice and lentil mix doesn't begin to burn or stick to the bottom.
8. Pour in most of the water or vegetable broth, throw in the cinnamon stick, cover with a lid, and bring the water to a boil.
9. Once the liquid is boiling, remove the lid, and add the rinsed rice.
10. Mix well, add salt to taste, and let it cook for another 15–20 minutes until both the rice and lentils are tender. Depending on the variety of rice and lentils, you may need to add the remaining water or it may need more or less time to cook. Adjust accordingly.
11. Turn off the heat, squeeze in some lemon juice to taste, and use a fork to fluff the mujadara.
12. Stir in the ground cumin and salt to taste.
13. Spoon the mujadara into a serving dish, top with the caramelized onions, and sprinkle with sumac, if using.
14. Garnish with fresh coriander or parsley, if desired.

Mexican Rice with Black Beans

While kitchari is often celebrated as the quintessential Ayurvedic dish combining rice, legumes, and spices, it's not the only way to enjoy this nourishing trio. Across cultures, rice and legumes are brought together in creative ways to deliver wholesome, comforting meals. This recipe is my Ayurvedic twist on the classic combination of rice and beans, infusing ancient wisdom with a modern, flavorful approach.

Prep time: 15 minutes
Cook time: 35 minutes
Serves 2 to 3

Ingredients
1 cup (6oz/170g) organic aged rice (sona masuri or basmati)
1 tablespoon ghee or extra virgin olive oil
1 small onion, finely chopped
2 cloves of garlic, minced
1 cup (6oz/175g) corn or other veggies (optional)
1 tomato (ideally boiled, peeled, and with pulp extracted – see page 282)
½ teaspoon ground cumin
½ teaspoon ground paprika
¼ teaspoon ground turmeric
¼ teaspoon ground cilantro (coriander)
½ teaspoon salt (adjust to taste)
2 cups (17fl oz/500ml) fresh vegetable broth or water
Fresh cilantro (coriander), chopped, to garnish (optional)
Lime wedges, to serve (optional)

For the black beans:
1 teaspoon ghee or olive oil
1 cup (6oz/170g) cooked black beans (see tip below)
½ teaspoon ground cumin
¼ teaspoon ground paprika
¼ teaspoon ground coriander
¼ teaspoon ground black pepper
Salt, to taste

Method

1. Rinse the sona masuri or basmati rice under cold water and set aside.
2. Heat the ghee or olive oil in a medium saucepan over medium heat.
3. Add the onion and sauté for about 3 to 4 minutes until translucent.
4. Add the minced garlic and cook for an additional 1 minute.
5. Add the corn or vegetables to the pan and cook for 4 to 5 minutes, stirring frequently.
6. Stir in the diced tomato and cook for 2 to 3 minutes, allowing the flavors to meld.
7. Add the rinsed rice, cumin, paprika, turmeric, cilantro (coriander), and salt. Stir well to coat the rice with the spices.
8. Pour in the vegetable broth or water. Bring to a boil.
9. Reduce the heat to low, cover, and simmer for about 15 minutes, or until the rice is cooked and the liquid is absorbed. Remove from heat and let it sit for 5 minutes before fluffing with a fork.
10. While the rice rests, prepare the black beans. In a small saucepan, heat the 1 teaspoon of ghee or olive oil over medium heat.
11. Add the cooked black beans, cumin, paprika, cilantro (coriander), black pepper, and salt. Stir well and cook

for about 5 minutes until heated through and the flavors are well combined.

12. Gently fold the spiced black beans into the cooked Mexican rice.

13. Transfer to serving dishes.

14. Garnish with fresh cilantro (coriander) and serve with lime wedges for squeezing, if desired.

Tip: To prepare the black beans, you will need ½ cup (3oz/85g) dried beans to yield 1 cup (6oz/170g) of cooked beans. Soak them in four times the volume of water overnight. Drain, then add them to a saucepan, cover with fresh water, and cook for 70 to 90 minutes, or cook them in a pressure cooker for 40 to 50 minutes, until tender.

Nidhi's Ayurvedic Kitchari with Buttermilk

This is a comforting one-pot traditional dish. This version simplifies the process and adds extra flavor while keeping it Ayurvedically balanced and fun to prepare. Enjoy your enhanced kitchari!

Prep time: 10 minutes (plus soaking the lentils and rice)
Cook time: 25 minutes
Serves 2 to 3

Ingredients

1 cup (7oz/200g) split mung lentils (soaked for 3 to 4 hours)
½ cup (3oz/85g) sona masuri rice (or pounded rice) (soaked for 30 minutes–1 hour)
1 tablespoon ghee (clarified butter), plus extra to serve
½ teaspoon mustard seeds
½ teaspoon cumin seeds
1 bay leaf
¼ teaspoon turmeric powder
A pinch of asafetida (hing) powder
1 small cinnamon stick
1 small piece of fresh ginger, peeled and minced
1 cup (about 6oz/175g) chopped or grated veggies of your choice (carrots, zucchini (courgette), bottle gourd/dudhi, etc.)
1 cup (2oz/ 60g) chopped spinach or any leafy greens (optional)
3 cups (26fl oz/750ml) boiling water
Himalayan salt, to taste
Juice of ½ lemon (optional, for added flavor)
Fresh cilantro (coriander), chopped, to garnish

Method

1. Rinse both the soaked mung lentils and sona masuri rice under cold water. Set aside.
2. Heat the 1 tablespoon of ghee in a large pot over medium heat.
3. Add the mustard seeds and wait until they start to pop.
4. Add cumin seeds, bay leaf, turmeric, asafetida, and the cinnamon stick. Sauté for 1 minute until fragrant.
5. Add the minced ginger and sauté for another minute.
6. Add the chopped or grated vegetables and the greens to the pot.
7. Sauté for about 5 minutes until the vegetables are slightly tender.
8. Add the rinsed rice and lentils to the pot. Stir to combine.
9. Pour in the boiling water.
10. Season with Himalayan salt.
11. Stir well and bring to a boil. Reduce heat to low–medium, cover and simmer until the water is absorbed and the rice and lentils are cooked (about 20 minutes), stirring occasionally.
12. Once cooked, switch off the heat and discard the cinnamon stick and bay leaf.
13. Add the lemon juice, if using, and stir gently.
14. Scoop a generous portion into bowls.
15. Top each serving with a dollop of ghee and stir until it emulsifies.
16. Garnish with fresh coriander.
17. Enjoy warm!

Tips: If there are any other spices you like to use, feel free to add them. I personally bloom (see page 191) nigella seeds and curry leaves in the ghee before adding the lentil and rice mix, if I am in the mood to play. I also like to add dried pomegranate seeds or pomegranate powder. All these ingredients support Agni and lower cholesterol, and also significantly enhance flavor.

If you want to make this in an Instant Pot, use 4 cups (35fl oz/1 liter) of water and cook on high pressure for 15 to 16 minutes. Allow a natural pressure release.

Ayurvedic Buttermilk

This is Ayurveda's answer to the microbiome-obsessed of the world. This is the OG gut replenisher. Yogurt brings in the warm and moist due to fermentation. When churned with water and paired with spices, this is the ultimate enhancer for your Agni. For best results, consume this drink 45 minutes to 1 hour after your lunch to aid digestion and refresh.

Prep time: 5 minutes
Serves 1

Ingredients

1 tablespoon plain yogurt (preferably organic and full-fat)
6 to 7 tablespoons room temperature water
Salt, to taste
¼ teaspoon roasted cumin seeds
¼ teaspoon grated fresh ginger
2 teaspoons chopped fresh cilantro (coriander) or mint (optional)
A pinch of black salt (kala namak) (optional, for added flavor)

Method

1. In a jug, combine the yogurt with the water. Adjust the amount of water based on your preferred consistency – more water for a thinner drink, less for a thicker consistency. Churn using a wooden hand churner or hand blender.
2. Add salt to taste.
3. Add the cumin seeds and the ginger.
4. Add the cilantro (coriander) or mint, if using.
5. Mix well.
6. Pour the drink into a glass and enjoy.

Bean and Sweet Potato Chili

Even non-Indian traditional foods have long adhered to the principles of "warm and moist," naturally aligning with what the body itself craves for balance and nourishment. This modern take, enriched with the subtle sweetness of sweet potatoes, offers a grounding, deeply nourishing, and irresistibly delicious twist on a time-honored tradition.

Prep time: 15 minutes (plus soaking the beans)
Cook time: 55 minutes–1 hour
Serves 2 to 3

Ingredients

⅓ cup (2¼oz/60g) dried black beans (soaked overnight)
⅓ cup (2¼oz/60g) dried pinto beans (soaked overnight)
½ cup (2oz/60g) sweet potatoes, diced
1 tablespoon ghee (or olive oil)
½ teaspoon cumin seeds
1 to 2 cloves of garlic, minced
½ onion, chopped (optional)
½ tomato, chopped (ideally boiled, peeled, and with pulp extracted – see tip below)
2 sticks of celery, chopped
1–2 carrots, peeled (if not organic) and chopped
1 bay leaf
½ teaspoon dried oregano
¼ teaspoon turmeric powder
¼ teaspoon ground coriander
¼ teaspoon chili powder (adjust to taste)
Salt, to taste

3 to 4 cups (26–35fl oz/750ml–1 liter) water or homemade
   vegetable broth
A squeeze of fresh lemon juice
Fresh cilantro (coriander) leaves, to garnish
1 small avocado, sliced (optional)

Method

1. Drain and rinse the soaked black beans and pinto beans
   and set aside.
2. Peel the sweet potatoes and dice into bite-sized pieces.
3. Heat 1 tablespoon of ghee or oil in a large saucepan.
4. Add the cumin seeds and sauté until they start to pop.
5. Add the minced garlic and cook for 1 minute until
   fragrant.
6. If using onion, add it and cook until translucent.
7. Add all the soaked beans to the pan.
8. Add the diced sweet potatoes, tomato, celery, carrots,
   bay leaf, dried oregano, turmeric, ground coriander, chili
   powder, and salt.
9. Stir to combine all the ingredients.
10. Pour in enough of the water or vegetable broth to cover
    the ingredients by about 1 inch (2.5cm). Cover with a
    lid and cook for 35–40 minutes, ensuring that the pan
    doesn't dry out. If needed, add extra water.
11. Turn off the stove when the beans are slightly
    overcooked. Mix well.
12. Check the seasoning and adjust with more salt or spices
    if needed and add a squeeze of lemon juice to taste.
13. Serve the stew hot, garnished with cilantro leaves and
    sliced avocados, if wished.

Tips: The solanine content in tomatoes – the alkaloid that
       makes it a nightshade and causes it to heat up your
       Inner Climate – can be reduced by boiling them. Throw
       the whole tomatoes in boiling water until the peel
       begins to crack. Remove the tomatoes and, when cool,

remove the peel with your fingers. Cut the body of the tomato from the center and remove and discard the pulp. *Voilà* – you're good to go!

You can also make this recipe in a pressure cooker. Rather than simmering on the stovetop, cook under pressure for about 30 minutes.

Ayurvedic Rice Pilaf with Raita

This Ayurvedic pilaf is one of my go-to lunch meals – rich in flavor yet light on the stomach. It strikes the perfect balance between nourishment and ease, offering a satisfying and wholesome dish that's easy to digest. Infused with spices that support digestion and vitality, this pilaf is a vibrant and delicious way to enjoy a balanced Ayurvedic meal.

Prep time: 15 minutes
Cook time: 30 minutes
Serves 2 to 3

Ingredients
For the pilaf:
1 cup (6oz/170g) organic sona masuri or basmati rice
1 tablespoon ghee or olive oil
½ teaspoon cumin seeds
1 small onion, finely chopped
2 cloves of garlic, minced
½ cup (about 2½oz/70g) mixed vegetables (such as finely diced carrots and bell peppers or peas), chopped
1 bay leaf
2 to 3 whole cloves
1 small cinnamon stick
½ teaspoon turmeric powder
½ teaspoon ground coriander
¼ teaspoon fennel seeds (optional)
2 cups (17fl oz/500ml) water
Salt, to taste
Fresh cilantro (coriander), to garnish (optional)

For the raita:
1 cup (8oz/225g) plain yogurt
½ cucumber, grated
1 tablespoon chopped fresh mint or cilantro (coriander) (optional)
¼ teaspoon ground cumin
Himalayan salt, to taste

Method

1. For the pilaf, rinse the rice under cold water until the water runs clear. Leave to soak in a bowl of fresh water for 10 minutes, then drain.
2. Heat the ghee or olive oil in a medium saucepan over medium heat.
3. Add the cumin seeds and cook until they start to pop.
4. Add the onion and cook for 3 to 4 minutes until translucent.
5. Stir in the garlic and cook for another 1 minute.
6. Add the chopped mixed vegetables, bay leaf, cloves, and cinnamon stick. Cook for 2 to 3 minutes.
7. Stir in the turmeric, coriander, and fennel seeds (if using). Cook for 1 minute to release the flavors.
8. Add the soaked and drained rice and stir to coat with the spices.
9. Pour in the water and add salt to taste.
10. Bring to a boil, then reduce the heat to low. Cover and simmer for 15 to 20 minutes, or until the rice is cooked and the water is absorbed.
11. Turn off the heat and let the pilaf sit for 5 minutes before fluffing with a fork.
12. To make the raita, combine the yogurt and grated cucumber in a bowl.
13. Stir in the chopped herbs (if using), the cumin, and a pinch of Himalayan salt.
14. Mix well.
15. Spoon the pilaf onto serving plates.
16. Serve with a side of raita and garnish with fresh cilantro (coriander) if desired.

Mung Lentil Stew with Fresh Herbs

Light, warm, and nourishing, green mung lentils are Ayurveda's answer to protein done right.

Prep time: 15 minutes, plus soaking the lentils
Cook time: 40 minutes–1 hour (depending on which lentils are used)
Serves 2 to 3

Ingredients

1 cup (6oz/170g) split mung lentils or whole mung lentils, rinsed
1 tablespoon ghee (or olive oil)
2 cloves of garlic, minced
1 stick of celery, chopped
½ onion, chopped
1 to 2 carrots, peeled (if not organic) and chopped
1 bay leaf
¼ teaspoon ground cumin
3–4 pinches of turmeric powder
Salt, to taste
2 cups (17fl oz/500ml) water if using split lentils OR 3 cups (26fl oz/750ml) if using whole mung lentils
A squeeze of lemon juice, to finish
Fresh parsley or cilantro (coriander), chopped, to garnish

Method

1. Soak the split lentils for 30 minutes prior to cooking. If using whole mung lentils, soak overnight or for a minimum of 2 hours, then drain.

2. In a pot, warm the ghee or olive oil and add the chopped garlic, celery, and onions. Cook for a few minutes until fragrant.
3. Add the carrots and cook for another few minutes until starting to soften.
4. Add the lentils, bay leaf, cumin, turmeric, and salt to taste, and mix well.
5. Add the water and let the stew simmer on a low–medium heat, half covered with a lid, until the lentils are tender – about 30 minutes if using split lentils or 45–50 minutes if using whole lentils. Stir every few minutes.
6. Ensure that the lentils are well-cooked before you turn off the heat. Add more boiling water if you like it less chunky, and some salt to taste.
7. Pour into serving bowls. Add a squeeze of lemon juice and garnish with cilantro (coriander) or parsley.

Ayurvedic Chickpea and Veggie Stew

This stew is a whole meal of itself. It's chunky, warm, and nourishing, and it's especially satisfying on a rainy or cold day. If you find chickpeas hard to digest, consider replacing them with whole mung beans instead.

Prep time: 10 minutes
Cook time: 40 minutes
Serves 2 to 3

Ingredients

1–2 teaspoons unrefined sesame oil or olive oil
1 bay leaf
2 teaspoons ginger–garlic paste
2 teaspoons ground cumin
1 teaspoon ground coriander
¼ teaspoon anise seed powder
1 teaspoon turmeric powder
¼–½ cup (2–4fl oz/60–120ml) vegetable stock (preferably homemade)
1 cup (about 6oz/175g) assorted chopped vegetables (e.g. carrots, celery, yams, leeks, red pepper)
½ cup (3oz/85g) dried chickpeas, soaked overnight and boiled (see tip below)
2.5 cups (22.5fl oz/625ml) water
A handful of baby spinach, roughly chopped
Salt, to taste
Crushed black pepper, to taste

Method

1. In a stockpot, warm the oil over medium heat.
2. Add the bay leaf and sauté for about 30 seconds.
3. Add the ginger–garlic paste and cook for 30 seconds.
4. Stir in the cumin, coriander, anise seed powder, and turmeric.
5. Sauté the spices for a few minutes, slowly adding the vegetable stock to release their flavors and create a fragrant base.
6. Add the chopped vegetables and drained chickpeas to the pot. Stir well to coat everything with the spices.
7. Pour in the water and bring to a simmer.
8. Cook for about 25 to 30 minutes, or until the vegetables are tender and the stew has a soup-like consistency. Keep a close eye on it and add more water, as needed.
9. Just before the end of the cooking time, add the chopped baby spinach. Stir until wilted but not overly mushy.
10. Season with salt and freshly crushed black pepper to taste.

Tip: To cook the chickpeas, soak them in four times the volume of water overnight. Drain, then add them to a saucepan, cover with fresh water, and cook for 30 minutes, or cook them in a pressure cooker for 20 minutes, until tender.

Simple Barley Stew

Barley can be a daily affair according to Ayurveda, yet it can be drying in the body for some as it's a scraper. This is also the reason why barley is used for weight loss, blood pressure, and high cholesterol. It also adds bulk to the diet, which is great for the bowels.

Prep time: 10 minutes
Cook time: 50 minutes
Serves 2 to 3

Ingredients
1 tablespoon olive oil or ghee
1 onion, chopped
1 potato, peeled and chopped
1 carrot, peeled (if not organic) and chopped
1 stalk of celery, chopped
1 cup (6½oz/185g) barley, washed
6 cups (48fl oz/1.4 liters) water
Salt and pepper, to taste
Chopped fresh herbs: ½ teaspoon parsley or ¼ teaspoon thyme (optional)

Method
1. Heat 1 tablespoon of olive oil or ghee in a pot.
2. Add the chopped onion, potato, carrot, and celery. Sauté the vegetables until they start to soften.
3. Add the barley to the pot.
4. Pour in the water.

5. Bring to a boil, then reduce the heat and simmer for 30 to 40 minutes, until the barley is tender and the stew has thickened.
6. Season with salt, pepper, and thyme or parsley, if using.
7. Stir well and enjoy your stew!

Favorite Vegetable Soup

My girls enjoy some variation of this soup on a daily basis. Sauté some celery, onions, and garlic and add any vegetables that you like to create your own different versions. And you can also sprinkle in your choice of seasonings or herbs. This recipe is super versatile!

Prep time: 10 minutes
Cook time: 25 minutes
Serves 2 to 3

Ingredients
1 tablespoon olive oil or ghee
1 celery stalk, chopped
1 small onion, diced
2 cloves of garlic, minced
1 medium carrot, peeled (if not organic) and chopped
1 small zucchini (courgette), chopped
1 bell pepper (any color), diced
2 cups (17fl oz/500ml) boiling water
Fresh or dried herbs (e.g. thyme, basil, parsley), to taste
Salt and pepper, to taste

Method
1. Heat the olive oil or ghee in a medium-sized pan over medium heat.
2. Add the celery, onion, garlic, carrot, zucchini (courgette), and bell pepper.
3. Sauté the vegetables, stirring occasionally, until they begin to soften and the onion is translucent, about 5–7 minutes.

4. Pour in the boiling water, ensuring the vegetables are covered.
5. Bring to a boil, then reduce the heat and let it simmer for about 10–15 minutes, or until the vegetables are tender.
6. Carefully transfer the mixture to a blender (or use an immersion (hand-held) blender) and blend until smooth.
7. If using a regular blender, blend in batches, and be cautious of hot splashes.
8. Return the blended soup to the pan.
9. Season with your choice of herbs and salt and pepper to taste.
10. Ladle the soup into bowls and serve hot.

APPENDIX 2
YOUR 21-DAY HEALING PROGRAM REVIEW AND MASTERY

Table 1: Review of the 21 Days

PRACTICE	BENEFITS EXPERIENCED	CHALLENGES	NOTES
Restore Your Relationship with Mealtimes			
Warm, Light Breakfast			
Heavy Lunch, Earlier Dinner			
Lighter Dinner			
No Cold Beverages			
Evaluate Your Relationship with Gadgets			
No Showering or Exercising with Food in Your Stomach			
Exercise			

YOUR 21-DAY HEALING PROGRAM REVIEW AND MASTERY

PRACTICE	BENEFITS EXPERIENCED	CHALLENGES	NOTES
Play with Your Caffeine Intake			
Sleep before 10pm			
Regulate Your Water Consumption			
Fats without Fear			
Spice It Up			
Adjust Your Shower Temperature			
Abhyanga Self-Love			
Nasya Your Nose			
Befriend Your Breath			
Oil Swishing			
Hair Abhyanga			
Foot Massage			
Gratitude and Radical Acceptance			

Table 2. 21-Day Healing Program Mastery

The practices marked with an asterisk* are non-negotiable and are important to maintain if you want to enjoy sustained transformation. You can choose to modify the intensity or number of days if you wish.

PRACTICE	YES/NO	X (DAYS PER WEEK), X (MINUTES PER DAY)	VACATIONS	BUSY PERIODS
Restore Your Relationship with Mealtimes				
Warm, Light Breakfast				
*Heavy Lunch, Earlier Dinner				
Lighter Dinner				
*No Cold Beverages				
Re-evaluate Your Relationship with Screens				
*No Showering or Exercising with Food in Your Stomach				
*Exercise				
Play with Your Caffeine Intake				

PRACTICE	YES/ NO	X (DAYS PER WEEK), X (MINUTES PER DAY)	VACATIONS	BUSY PERIODS
Sleep before 10pm				
*Regulate Your Water Consumption				
*Fats without Fear				
*Spice It Up				
Adjust Your Shower Temperature				
Abhyanga Self-Love				
Nasya Your Nose				
Befriend Your Breath				
Oil Swishing				
Hair Abhyanga				
Foot Massage				
Gratitude and Radical Acceptance				

APPENDIX 3
YOUR WELL-BEING CHART

Use this chart as a template to monitor your bowel movements, sleep, period, mood, and weight during the course of the 21-day healing program and to record any changes you observe.

	Week One	Week Two	Week Three
Bowel movements			
Sleep			
Period			
Mood			
Weight			

APPENDIX 4
SEASONS

Season	Body Adaptations	Diet	Exercise	Sleep
Winter	Pores constrict; Agni increases; brown fat and thyroid activity rise.	High-calorie, grounding foods with good fats, whole grains, root vegetables, nuts, seeds.	Generous workouts; body doesn't tire easily.	Longer sleep duration; earlier bedtime.
Spring	Mucus melts, humidity rises; Agni weakens.	Lighter, drier foods (barley, roasted grains, honey). Gradual fruit intake.	Moderate intensity to release fluids.	Avoid daytime naps to prevent sluggishness.
Summer	Open pores; appetite decreases, thirst rises.	Lighter, cooling foods (watery broths, rice, fruits in moderation).	Light yoga or mild activity; avoid heavy exercise.	Afternoon naps allowed to preserve moisture.
Fall	Cooling temperatures; body prepares for winter.	Transition to grounding foods; cooked fruits (e.g. apples, pears).	Moderate exercise; gentle transition from summer's intensity.	Gradually shift to longer sleep hours in preparation for winter.

APPENDIX 5
LIFE SEASONS

Life Phase	Description	Diet	Exercise	Sleep
Childhood (Spring)	Growth phase; body is wet and tender, with high growth hormone.	Light, nourishing, and warm foods (e.g. rice, almonds, ghee, vegetables); avoid overfeeding, processed foods, refined sugars, and cold beverages.	Prioritize movement over exercise; avoid muscle-heavy routines and high-stretch activities like yoga.	Deep sleep is crucial for growth and nervous system development.
Youth (Summer)	Transformation phase; estrogen and progesterone fuel growth and warmth.	Balanced diet with good fats and spices; eat at appropriate times to maintain inner flame and vitality.	Exercise between 6-10am, include good fats in diet; exercise to half capacity.	Balance solar (exercise) with lunar (rest); incorporate oil massage, meditation, silent time, and screen-free periods.
Middle Age (Fall)	Beginning of body's drying phase; estrogen and progesterone fluctuate.	Warm, moist foods (e.g. avocado, sweet potatoes, coconut, cooked grains, ghee); include oil massage to nourish skin.	Yoga for flexibility and strength; gentle cardio (like dance) that supports joint health and mental well-being.	Meditation and pranayama can support repair work; avoid daytime napping and excessive screen time.
Old Age (Winter)	Body becomes dry and cold, with low estrogen and progesterone. A time for self-discovery and peace.	Light broths, dates, almonds, rice, and soups to reduce bloating; lower fat and protein intake for ease of digestion.	Gentle activities like Pilates, yoga, and walks in nature; avoid high-impact exercises; incorporate navel oiling with sesame or almond oil.	Deepen meditation practice, reflect and release; allow for light naps (20-40 minutes) in the day; practice forgiveness and gratitude for a peaceful mind.

NOTES

1   Marilyn Hair and Jon Sharpe, "Fast Facts About the Human Microbiome," The Center for Ecogenetics and Environmental Health, University of Washington, https://depts.washington.edu/ceeh/downloads/FF_Microbiome.pdf.

2   Harrison Wein, ed., "Your Microbes and You: The Good, Bad and Ugly," NIH News in Health website, https://newsinhealth.nih.gov/2012/11/your-microbes-you#:~:text=The%20microbiome%20actually%20provides%20more,is%20to%20help%20with%20digestion.

3   Maddie Burakoff, "Science explains how cooking food and gathering for feasts made us human," *Los Angeles Times*, Nov. 21, 2022, https://www.latimes.com/science/story/2022-11-21/how-cooking-food-and-gathering-for-feasts-made-us-human.

4   "Baking sourdough bread to boost your inner ecosystem," Dr. Gabrielle Cremer Consulting website, Apr. 4, 2020, www.cremerconsulting.com/en/baking-sourdough-bread-to-boost-your-inner-ecosystem/.

5   "Stomach Acid Secretion," Science Direct website, www.sciencedirect.com/topics/biochemistry-genetics-and-molecular-biology/stomach-acid-secretion#:~:text=These%20investigators%20described%20a%20peak,the%20absence%20of%20meal%20stimulation.

6   HRNews Wire, "Yes, drinking more water may help you lose weight," Hub at Work, John Hopkins University website, Jan 15, 2020, https://hub.jhu.edu/at-work/2020/01/15/focus-on-wellness-drinking-more-water/.

7   R. Taléns-Visconti et al, "Intranasal Drug Administration in Alzheimer-Type Dementia: Towards Clinical Applications," *Pharmaceutics*, May 3, 2023; 15(5):1399.

8   P. Saha et al, "Intranasal nanotherapeutics for brain targeting and clinical studies in Parkinson's disease," *J Control Release*. Jun 2023; 358:293–318.

9   M.R. Farag et al, "The Toxicological Aspects of the Heat-Borne Toxicant 5-Hydroxymethylfurfural in Animals: A Review," *Molecules*, Apr 22, 2020; 25(8):1941.

ABOUT THE AUTHOR

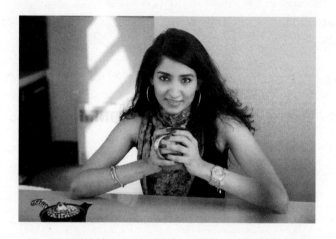

Nidhi Bhanshali Pandya is a certified Ayurvedic Doctor, a speaker, and creator of the Inner Climate Method®—a transformative approach that blends ancient Vedic widom with modern science. Based in New York City, she brings 15 years of expertise and a lifelong immersion in Ayurveda, inspired by her grandfather, a revered Ayurvedic healer in India.

Formally trained for over five years at a traditional Gurukulam-type institution, Nidhi excels in distilling complex ancient scriptures into practical, modern-day tools. Her passion lies in empowering people to cultivate self-awareness, live intuitively, and achieve mind-body balance. Through her globally taught Inner Climate Method® and now her book

Your Body Already Knows, she helps readers and students harness their intuition and innate wisdom to achieve sustainable health and well-being, while providing a systematic guide to reset their gut, hormones, sleep, and mood.

As a faculty member at the Shakti School, a contributor to leading publications, and the creator of a course on Commune, Nidhi bridges the gap between traditional Ayurvedic teachings and contemporary lifestyles.

Her TEDx talk and teachings have inspired audiences worldwide, proving that vibrant health and happiness are attainable for modern women everywhere.